Kid Fitness

KID FITNESS

Radu Teodorescu
with Brooks Roberts

Seaview Books
New York

Manufactured in the United States of America.

FIRST EDITION

Trade distribution by Simon and Schuster
A Division of Gulf + Western Corporation
New York, New York 10020

Library of Congress Cataloging in Publication Data

Teodorescu, Radu, 1944-
      Kid fitness.

      1. Motor ability in children.   2. Exercise for chil-
dren.   I. Roberts, Brooks, joint author.   II. Title.
RJ133.T46   613.7′1   79-12680
ISBN 0-87223-534-3

CONTENTS

2053836

CONTENTS

Kid Fitness

INTRODUCTION

An organized daily exercise period for your child? Is that really necessary? After observing the physical activities of many American children, from infancy to preteens, I am convinced it is. In cities and suburbs, school buses provide door-to-door service; twice-weekly gym classes are usually devoted to games that offer entertainment but little real exercise; playgrounds often resemble a subway train at rush hour.

Therefore, if you want your son or daughter to enjoy a graceful, strong, healthy body, you will have to assume the responsibility personally, just as you do in providing nourishing food and suitable clothes, and encouraging hygienic habits.

There is a difference, however. This can be one of the most rewarding responsibilities of your life, both emotionally and physically. It is an emotional experience because you will be engaged in a mutually enjoyable one-to-one activity with your child. It is a physical experience because you will be doing the exercises with your child—that's a requirement—and your body will benefit as well as the child's.

But in order to maintain an exercise program, day after day and year after year, you must be completely convinced of its value. Let me explain to you why I am.

First, I believe that we all need healthy, active bodies to throw off the strain and tension of our sedentary lives—early years spent over books, later years at office desks. The Romans recognized the unity of body and mind with the ideal of *mens sana in corpore sano*—a sound mind in a healthy body. Every jogger who tells you how relaxed and invigorated he or she feels after running a few miles is rediscovering that truth.

It is also true that when we look good we tend to feel better about ourselves, and thus be more self-confident. This enables us to face new challenges and relate more easily to people. I don't think it's an accident that the majority of successful people have straight, trim bodies that they keep in shape.

Exercising is particularly important for children between the ages of six months and eleven years, because this period is characterized by explosive growth. Arms and legs are too long for the body, stomachs too big, and chests too narrow. Muscles are weak, and nervous systems are still developing. A daily exercise program can help children in these formative years by building stronger, better coordinated bodies. They will enter the turbulent teens with more self-confidence, more likely to excel in organized sports, at ease with their maturing bodies.

Are systematic, supervised exercises necessary? Isn't ordinary play with other children enough? I'm all for your child running and jumping, throwing and climbing with other children, but in our crowded, spectator-oriented world, those activities don't take place often enough. And, secondly, children's bodies need different exercises during different stages. That's why this book is divided into four age groups, with each set of exercises based on the ones that preceded it. They progress from the known to the unknown, from the easy to the complex, and therefore must be done in an organized, methodical way.

Perhaps as a result of my European upbringing, I also feel that organization and discipline are valuable elements in children's lives. Daily exercises, while building strong bodies and increasing self-confidence, also serve to teach children that improvement is achieved only as a result of hard work—a lesson that will be useful throughout their lives.

It is easy to understand why exercises for children up to three or four years must be supervised by a parent, but you may wonder if it is necessary past that time. Yes, it is.

You'll find that children require constant inspiration, as well as constant instruction, to perform these exercises both correctly and enthusiastically. For most of the years covered by this book, you'll have to exercise right along with your child, providing the essential example to be imitated. Your voice not only sets the rhythm, its brightness and vigor set the tone for the session.

Safety is another reason supervision is needed. For example, it's up to you to make sure that warm-ups are performed properly, to reduce the chance of a pulled muscle later. And since an occasional fall is practically inevitable for awkward young bodies, you should make sure that the exercise area is cleared and that the floor isn't slippery.

My one precaution is that you discuss this exercise program with your pediatrician and get medical approval. Some children have special needs, which the doctor can point out. At subsequent medical checkups you can also get an idea of your progress.

If there is only one thought I can leave with you, let it be this: Your child will succeed in getting the benefits from these exercises only if you enjoy doing them. If you view them as pleasurable periods of exertion, your child will, too.

Chapter I

THE WHERE, WHEN, AND HOW OF EXERCISING WITH YOUR CHILD

Before you begin your exercise program, there are a few simple rules and guidelines that you should be familiar with. It is important to follow them closely. Here's what you need to know:

What equipment is required?

None. All you need is a clear floor space eight or ten feet square. A carpeted area is preferable; but if that's not available, spread oversize beach towels for exercises that involve lying down. Open a window for fresh air. If you have a yard, it's fun to exercise outdoors in good weather.

When is the best time to work out?

Whatever time best fits your child's schedule and yours—a time when neither of you will feel rushed. Exercises shouldn't be done less than an hour before or two hours after meals, to avoid interfering with digestion. It is also preferable to have your sessions at the same time every day, because establishing such a pattern will cause the body automatically to provide extra adrenaline beforehand, in anticipation of the workout.

How often should we work out?

A child from six months to one year should be exercised at least five times a week. Before the bath seems to be a good time.

For children one to two years old, the minimum should be four sessions a week.

From that age on, exercises should be done at least three times a week. Try to schedule them for days when the child doesn't have gym class in school.

What should we wear?

Shorts and T-shirts are fine; mothers and daughters may prefer leotards. Exercising indoors can be done in bare feet, but wear sneakers outdoors.

How should we begin?

Start by doing just one exercise from each group for the arms, neck, etc. Concentrate on achieving a smooth rhythm and correct execution, checking your child's movements against the photos. Repeat each exercise four times. Every other day, add another exercise from each group, until you are doing all of them in your daily sessions.

After a month, do each exercise six times; after eight months, graduate to eight times, unless a different number is suggested for a specific exercise.

Tips for the teacher

1. Memorize beforehand the exercises you are going to introduce. This makes for a smoother lesson.

2. At the start, give the exercises in the same order. This will make them easier to remember.

3. Be quick to notice and correct any errors in execution before they become ingrained habits.

4. After strenuous exercises, or if you notice your child is breathing hard, take time out for

deep breathing. "Arms up" (from the sides): Inhale. "Arms down": Exhale.

5. Slow the pace for the final few minutes of the session to allow the child's body to calm down.

6. Make a point of remarking on how well an exercise was performed, or on any improvements you see.

7. Note how *your* performance of the exercises is improving.

Chapter II

AGE SIX MONTHS TO TWO YEARS

At six months most children are almost helpless, able to sit up only with support, to grasp objects but release them only with difficulty. In a few more months a child can sit up alone and then crawl, and by a year he or she may discard crawling for toddling. Before they are two, they are constantly running, climbing stairs, playing chase games.

The purpose of the exercises for this group is both to ease and to speed the tremendous transition the child is making from a sedentary infant to an active, if clumsy, biped. Strengthening muscles improves the coordination needed for all these exciting new activities, and there is strong evidence that physical activity helps the development of the nervous system. Certainly the ability

to walk gives the child confidence and the opportunity to explore and learn from the environment.

Because of the great changes in physical activities that take place during this period, and the different muscles used, I have developed one set of exercises for the child between six months and one year, another for the child between one and two years. A certain amount of care must be taken when you are doing the exercises for the child. Because your child's nervous system is still incomplete, the reaction to pain is slow, so it is up to you to work gently and cautiously.

Again, please remember that your child is extremely sensitive to your moods. If you approach these exercises without any enthusiasm, your child may decide they're unpleasant. If you regard them as another reason to hold and play with your child, the exercise period can be a time of love and laughter for both of you.

WARM-UP

Until the child is walking, the body is prepared for exercises by a massage, which is administered from the extremities in toward the trunk. With the child lying facedown, start at the feet and, with long, gentle strokes, rub upward along the legs and back, helping the blood return to the heart.

Next, start at the hands and rub the arms, shoulders, and back. Repeat with a slightly deeper massage to the same areas, using the fingertips to describe circles. For variety, you can have your fingertips imitate raindrops. Then roll your child over on the back and finish the warm-up with a gentle massage of the chest, not the stomach. All of this should take three or four minutes.

Your eighteen-month-old child may enjoy such a massage before exercising, but usually a little tickling is enough to get the circulation speeded up—and it also sets a good tone for the exercise session.

FOR THE ARMS

(The purpose of these exercises is to stretch—very gently—muscles which the baby naturally tends to keep contracted. They can be done with the child lying down or sitting up, whichever works best for both of you.)

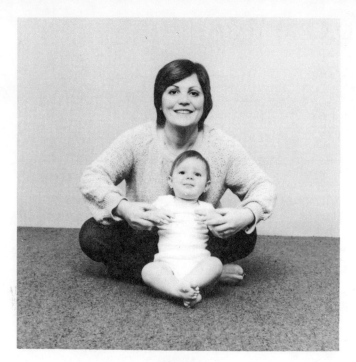

Figure 1

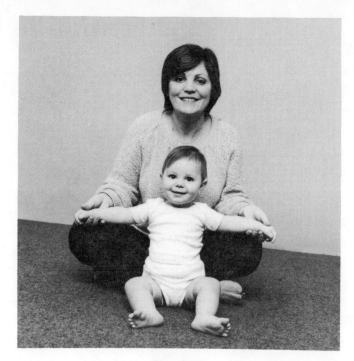

Figure 2

1. Holding the forearms, gently bend and straighten the arms out to the sides. *(See figures 1 and 2.)*

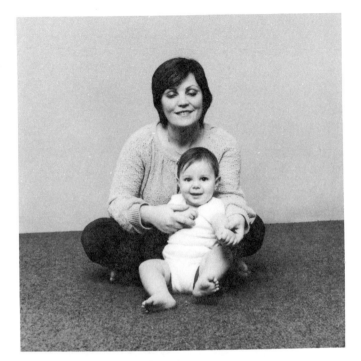

Figure 3

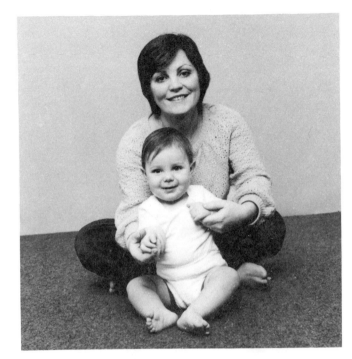

Figure 4

2. Holding the forearms, alternately bend and straighten each arm in front, as in a piston movement. *(See figures 3 and 4.)*

19

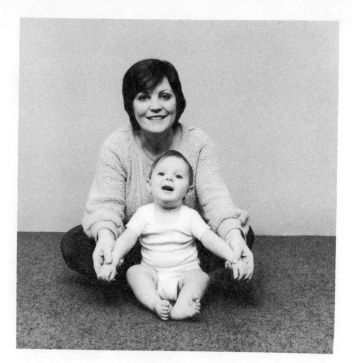

Figure 5

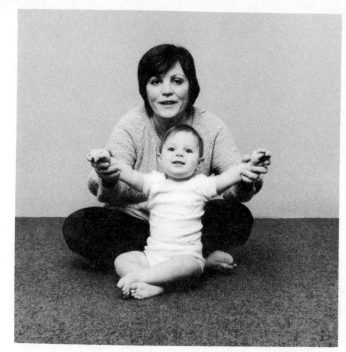

Figure 6

3. Hold the baby's arms by the wrists, extended in front. Move the arms in opposing circles, first one direction, then the other. *(See figures 5 and 6.)*

FOR THE TRUNK

(These stretching and strengthening exercises should be done with the child lying on the back, except for number 4.)

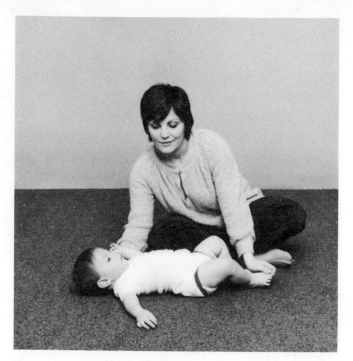

Figure 7

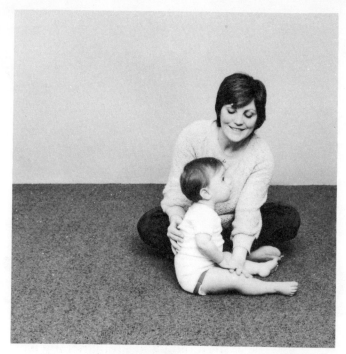

Figure 8

1. Put your arm behind the back, supporting the head. Encourage and help the child to sit up, then lower the child back to the floor. *(See figures 7 and 8.)*

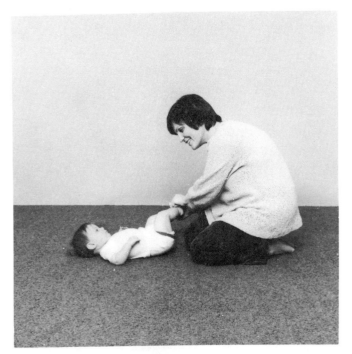

Figure 9

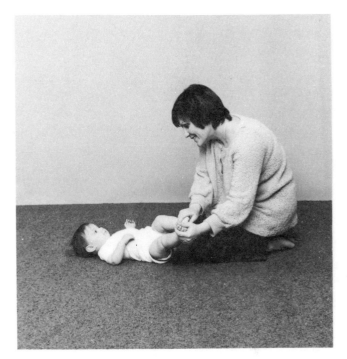

Figure 10

2. Bend the legs at the knees and tilt them together from side to side. *(See figures 9 and 10.)*

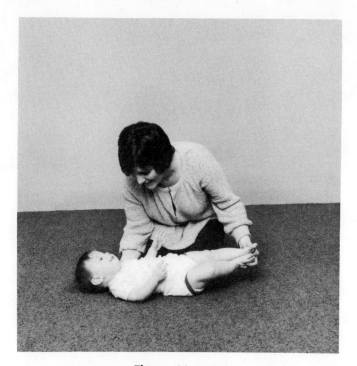

Figure 11

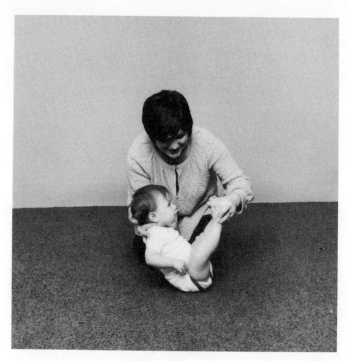

Figure 12

3. Put one hand under the back, the other under the heels, and raise them both at the same time. *(See figures 11 and 12.)*

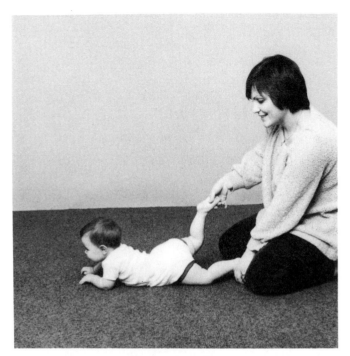

Figure 13

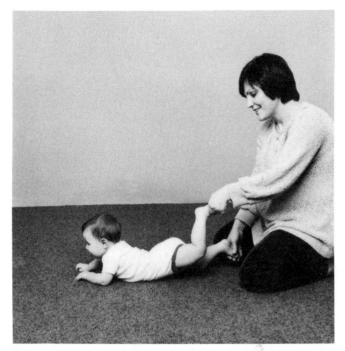

Figure 14

4. With the child lying on the stomach, raise the right leg, then the left. *(See figures 13 and 14.)*

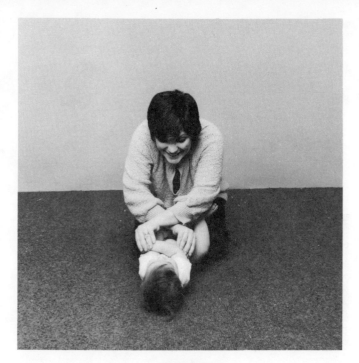

Figure 15

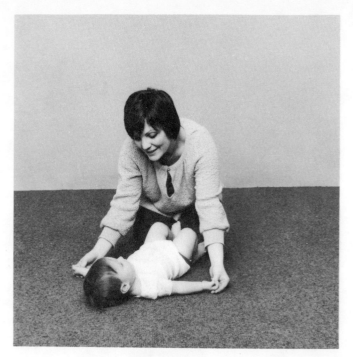

Figure 16

5. With the child lying on the back, cross arms over chest and then open them in a scissors movement. *(See figures 15 and 16.)*

FOR THE LEGS

(This set of exercises will help your child get ready for that great event—the first step.)

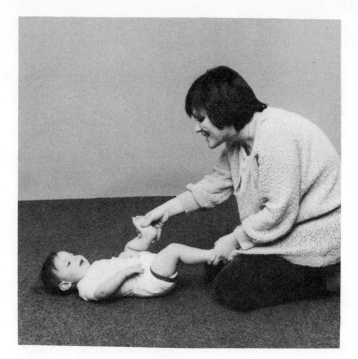

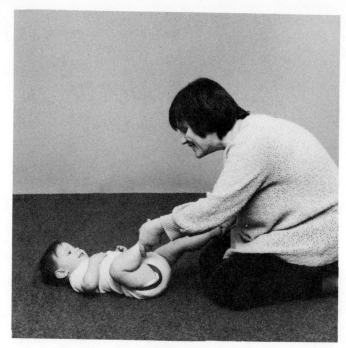

Figure 17   **Figure 18**

1. With the child on the back, hold the feet, "bicycle" them forward, then backward. *(See figures 17 and 18.)*

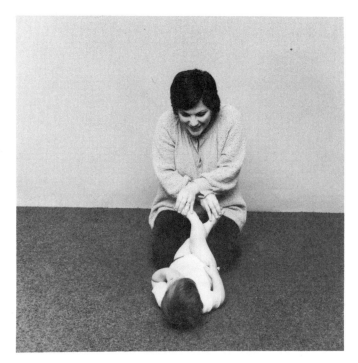

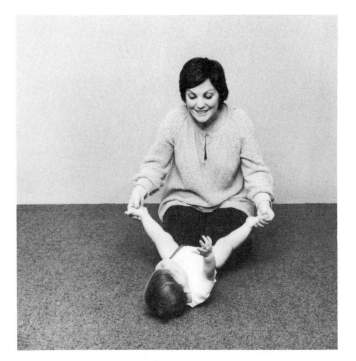

Figure 19   **Figure 20**

2. With the child on the back, take the legs by the ankles and cross them back and forth. *(See figures 19 and 20.)*

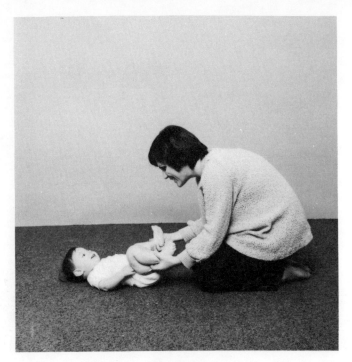

Figure 21

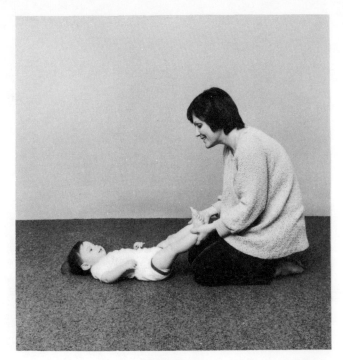

Figure 22

3. With the child on the back, grasp legs by the ankles and bend legs to the side, then straighten. *(See figures 21 and 22.)*

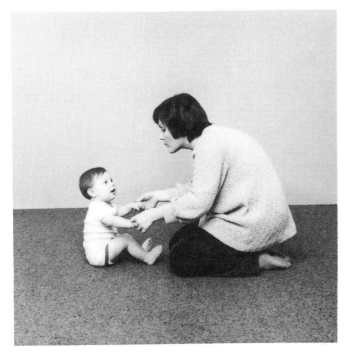

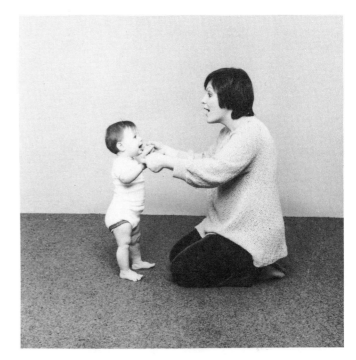

Figure 23 **Figure 24**

4. With the child in a sitting position, hold his or her hands and raise to a standing position. *(See figures 23 and 24.)*

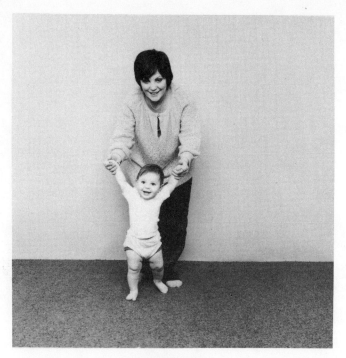

Figure 25

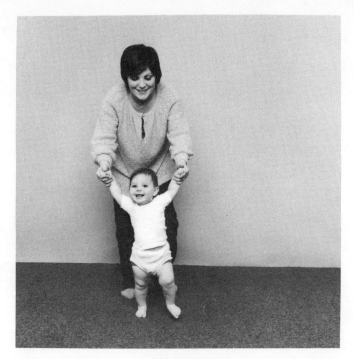

Figure 26

5. Support the child in a standing position by holding the arms and help him or her to walk. *(See figures 25 and 26.)*

FOR THE ARMS

(Our goal again is to stretch those muscles that tend to be held in a contracted position.)

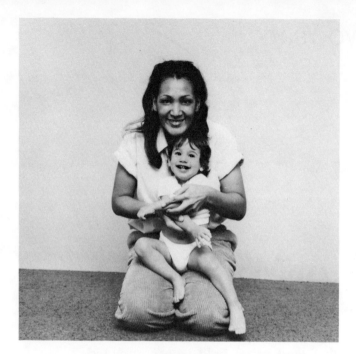

Figure 27

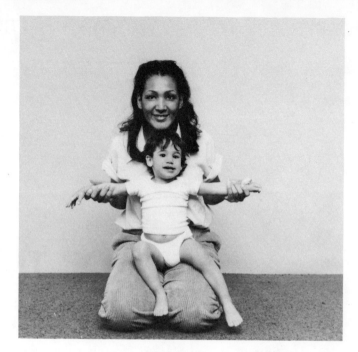

Figure 28

1. With the child lying or sitting on your lap, cross the arms in front and swing up and out in large circles. Then do this in the opposite direction. *(See figures 27 and 28.)*

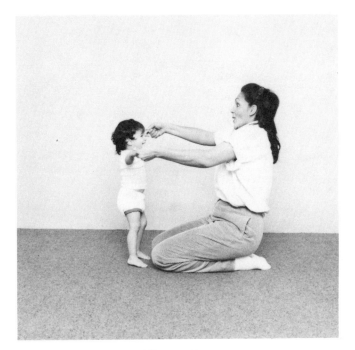

Figure 29

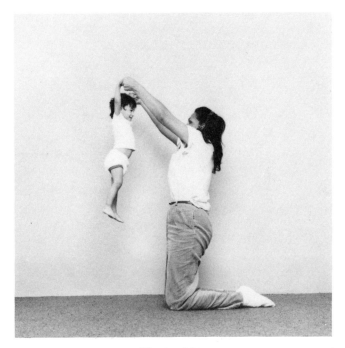

Figure 30

2. With the child standing, let him or her grasp your index fingers. Raise your hands so the child's weight is stretching the arms. *(See figures 29 and 30.)*

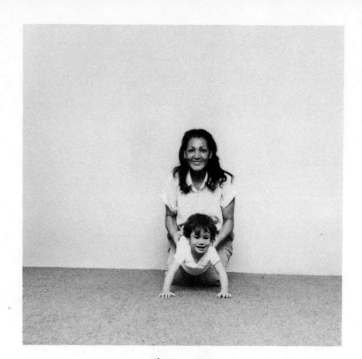

Figure 31

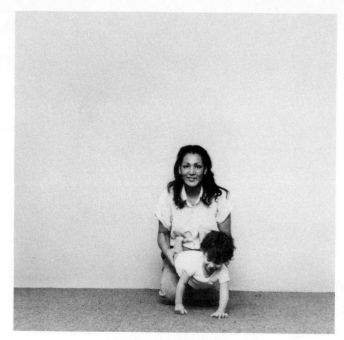

Figure 32

3. With the child lying facedown, lift the upper legs so the child pushes down with the hands for support. *(See figures 31 and 32.)*

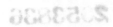

FOR THE NECK

(At this age the neck muscles are weak, so you must perform these exercises with your hands on each side of the child's head, holding gently but securely.)

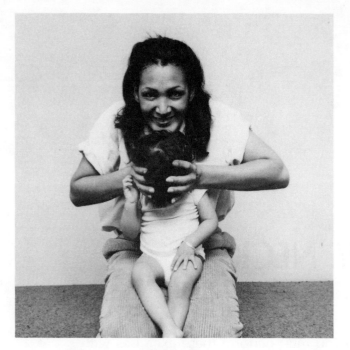

Figure 33

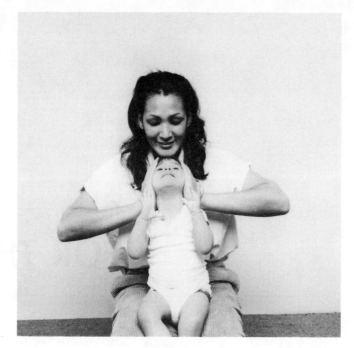

Figure 34

1. Bend the head down toward the chest and then up. *(See figures 33 and 34.)*

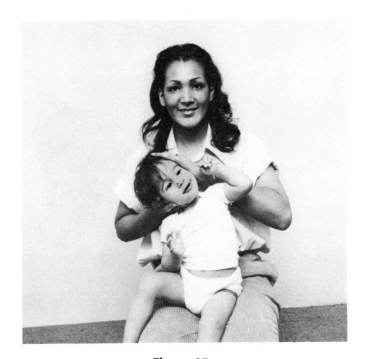

Figure 35

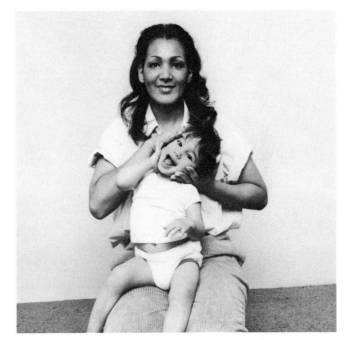

Figure 36

2. Bend the head to the right, then to the left. *(See figures 35 and 36.)*

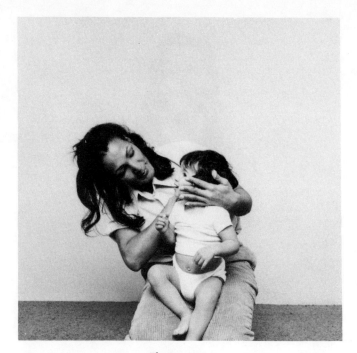

Figure 37

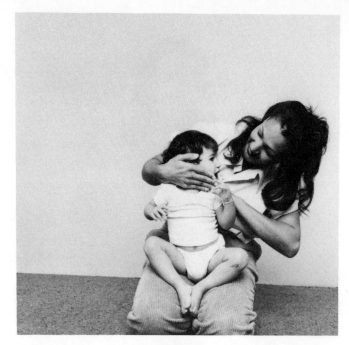

Figure 38

3. Turn the head to the right, then to the left. *(See figures 37 and 38.)*

FOR THE TRUNK

(Although children of this age spend most of their waking hours "exercising," the following movements use muscles that require special attention.)

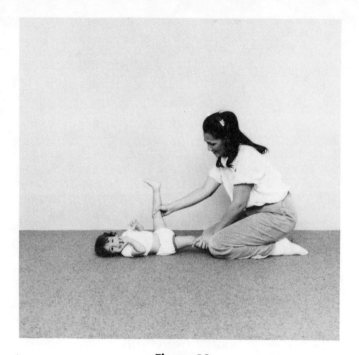

Figure 39

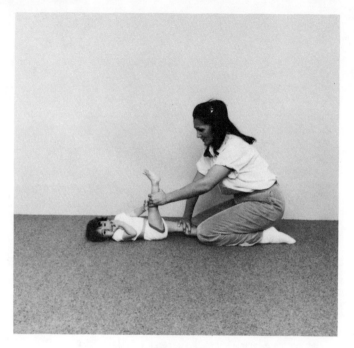

Figure 40

1. With the child lying on the back, hold the legs so they are straight and scissor them forward and back. *(See figures 39 and 40.)*

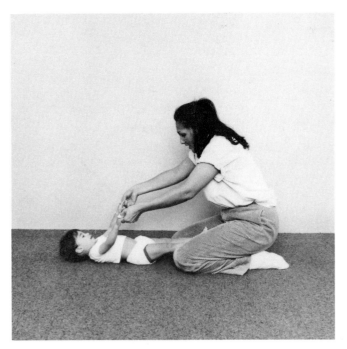

Figure 41

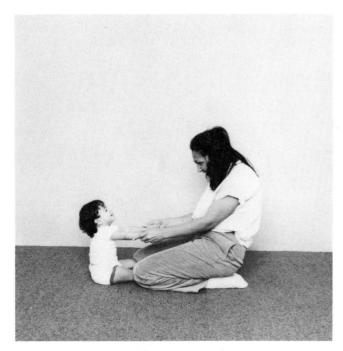

Figure 42

2. With the child lying on the back, let him or her grasp your index fingers. Help raise the child to a sitting position, then lower. *(See figures 41 and 42.)*

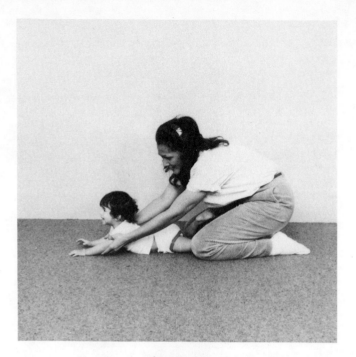

Figure 43

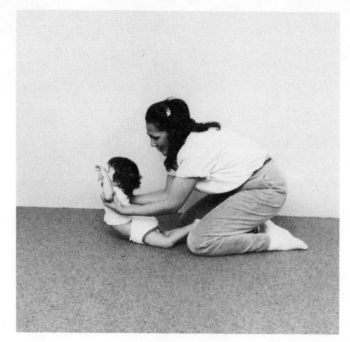

Figure 44

3. With the child lying facedown and arms stretched overhead, hold the elbows and raise gently, then lower. *(See figures 43 and 44.)*

FOR THE LEGS

(Your child is either walking or about to start, and these exercises will make it easier.)

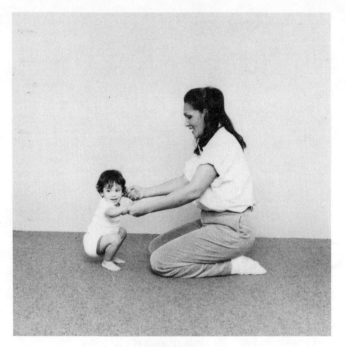

Figure 45

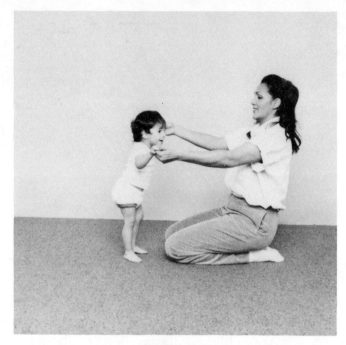

Figure 46

1. With the child standing and holding your index fingers for support, raise and lower your hands so the legs are bent and straightened. *(See figures 45 and 46.)*

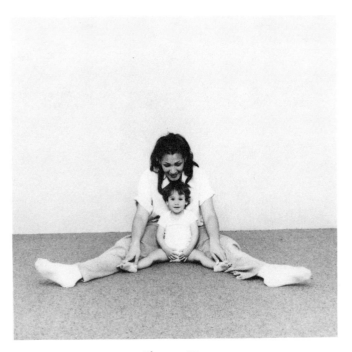

Figure 47

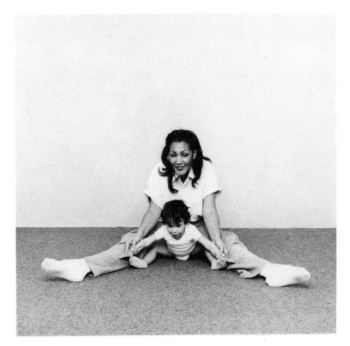

Figure 48

2. With the child in a sitting position, legs apart, stretch arms toward the toes. *(See figures 47 and 48.)*

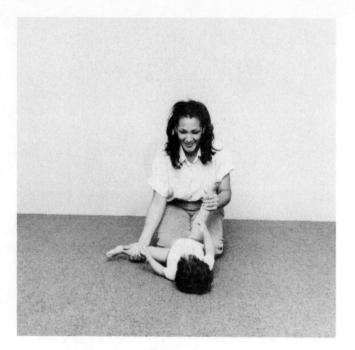

Figure 49

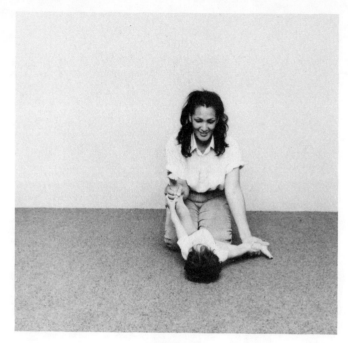

Figure 50

3. With the child on the back, grasp ankles and hold legs straight up. Bring one leg down to the floor at the side and up, then the other. *(See figures 49 and 50.)*

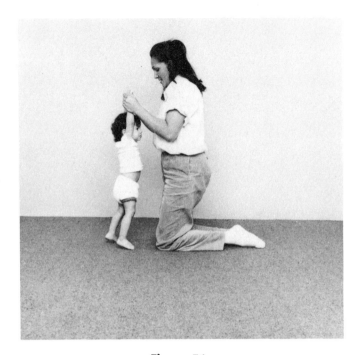

Figure 51

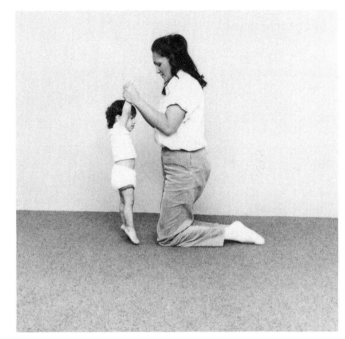

Figure 52

4. As the child stands and is held by the hands, he or she will make very small jumps with encouragement and a little lift. *(See figures 51 and 52.)*

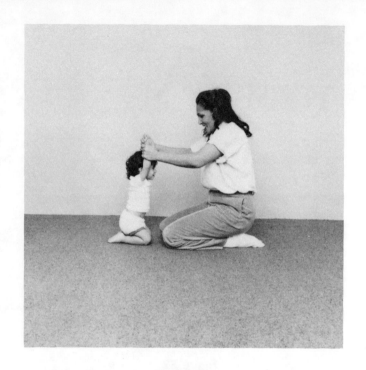

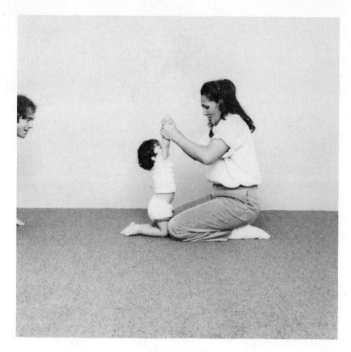

Figure 53   **Figure 54**

5. With the child sitting back on the heels, hold by the arms and raise to a kneeling position, then down. *(See figures 53 and 54.)*

Chapter III

AGE TWO TO FIVE

At two your child is still part infant, active but awkward, with underdeveloped motor coordination. Three years from now, with help from you and nature, he or she will stand erect instead of with that infantile lean, and will walk and run gracefully instead of toddling with arms extended.

This, then, is a period with tremendous potential for growth, yet it also presents some problems. For one, the parent must keep in mind that even an energetic two- or three-year-old has underdeveloped muscles, a fragile skeleton, poor coordination, and brief endurance; exercises have to be carefully regulated to the child's abilities. Even so, at this age many children may not be able to perform all of the prescribed exercises precisely. However, all efforts are helping their growth.

Secondly, children during these years experience changes in their emotional development. Around their second and third birthdays, children tend to be cooperative and show noticeable improvement in terms of motor skills. But at two and a half and three and a half, you may find your child balking at the established routine and actually losing some of the coordination previously acquired.

Great patience is necessary to get through these difficult periods. Keep the lessons very elastic, and jump to a new exercise before boredom sets in. Take advantage of the fact that your child is now old enough to understand simple explanations of why he or she is exercising—he will be able to climb stairs, or run faster to meet daddy. Explain that he is learning to jump like a rabbit, stretch like a cat—or compare his feats to those of his favorites on television or in books. It won't always be easy, but your job is to make your child enjoy the exercises. Your goal of good posture and graceful movements, which you can achieve by the end of these years, is worth the effort.

WARM-UP

Help your child get tuned up for the exercise session with a lively, brief (three- or four-minute) warm-up period. Walk on tiptoe, then on the heels. Run in place, forward and backward, then run while keeping the knees straight. Jump with legs out to the sides, then jump and kick them up to the rear. Jump with one leg forward, one back, and alternate. With hands on hips and legs apart, bend four times to each side, then four times forward. Rotate the arms at shoulder level. With legs apart, swing arms up, arching back, then reach forward to the floor.

Switch to another activity as soon as the child slows down or signals otherwise that boredom might be setting in.

FOR THE ARMS

(These exercises are designed to develop strength, elasticity, speed, and coordination.)

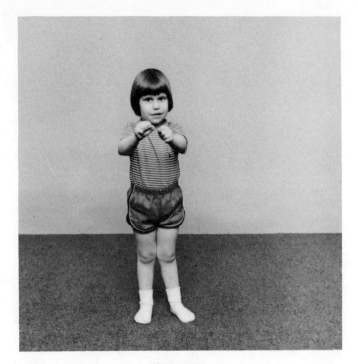

Figure 55

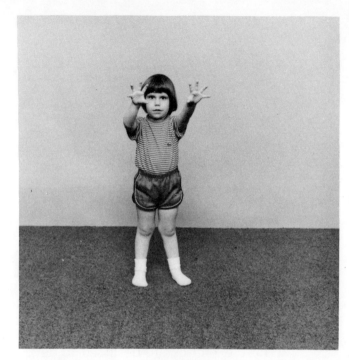

Figure 56

1. Stand with legs apart and arms in front at shoulder level. Make fists and then extend fingers as quickly as possible. *(See figures 55 and 56.)*

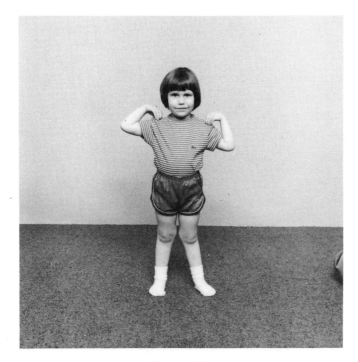

Figure 57

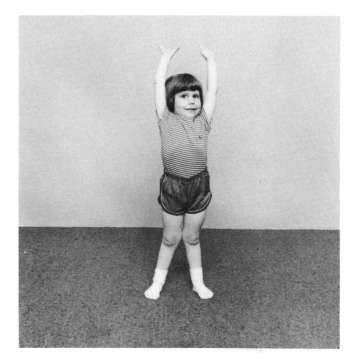

Figure 58

2. Stand with legs apart. Bring hands to shoulders, then overhead, back to shoulders, and down. *(See figures 57 and 58.)*

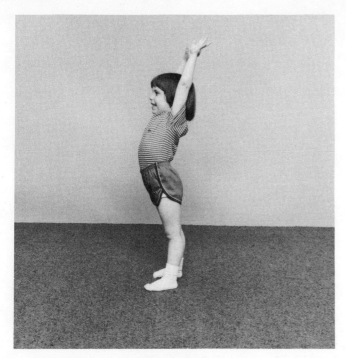

Figure 59

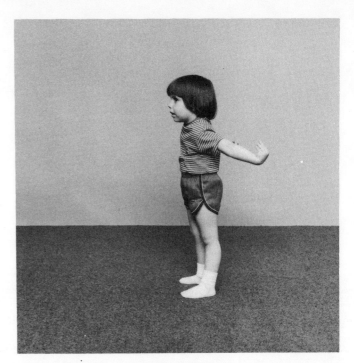

Figure 60

3. Starting with arms at sides, swing them forward and overhead, then down and as far back as possible. *(See figures 59 and 60.)*

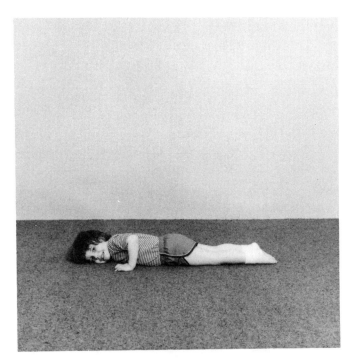

Figure 61

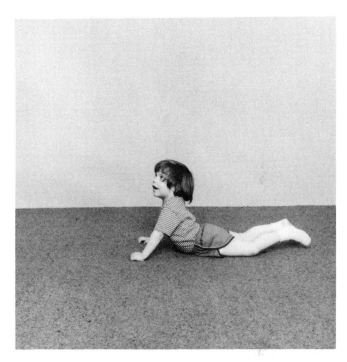

Figure 62

4. Lie prone on the floor, with palms under shoulders. Push up chest, raising head back, then down. *(See figures 61 and 62.)*

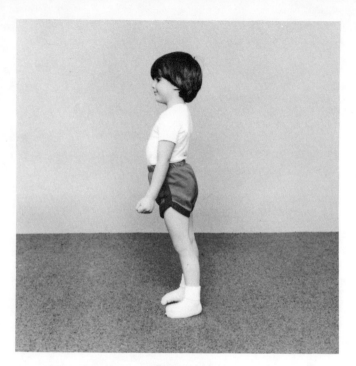

Figure 63

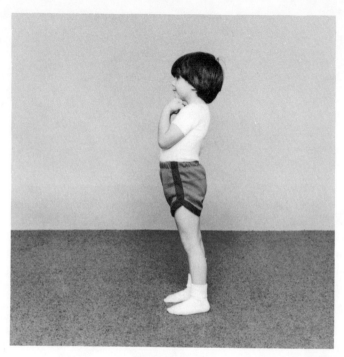

Figure 64

5. Stand with fists at sides. Bring fists forward to touch shoulders, then down to sides. *(See figures 63 and 64.)*

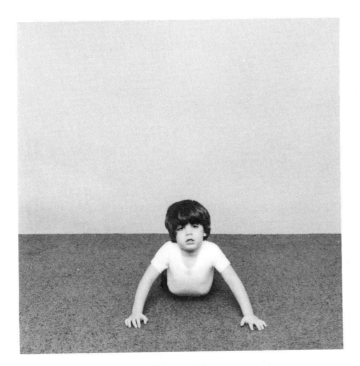

Figure 65

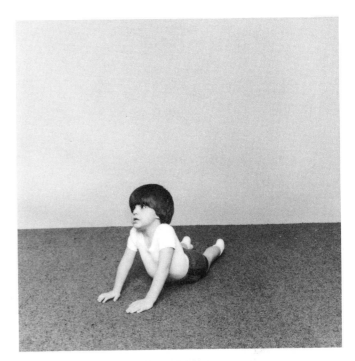

Figure 66

6. Support body on toes and hands on floor, with arms straight. "Walk" hands six steps to the right, then to the left. *(See figures 65 and 66.)*

FOR THE NECK

(A strong, straight neck is an essential element of correct posture. Since the neck isn't going to add any more articulations, these same exercises should also be used for the five-to-eight-year-old group. They can, of course, be done more vigorously as the child gets older. Do them sitting or standing, with feet apart and hands on hips.)

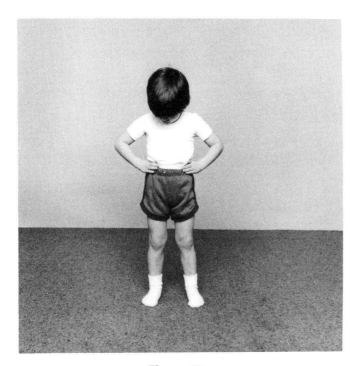

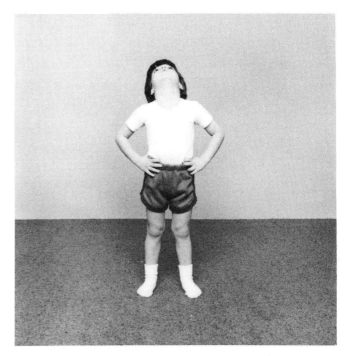

Figure 67   **Figure 68**

1. Bend head down to the chest and then arch backward. *(See figures 67 and 68.)*

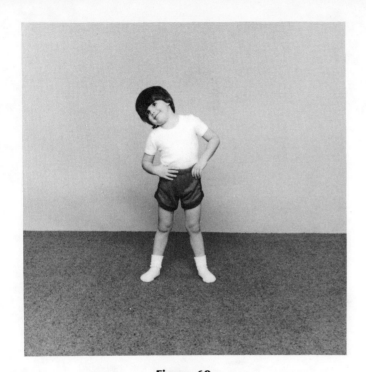

Figure 69

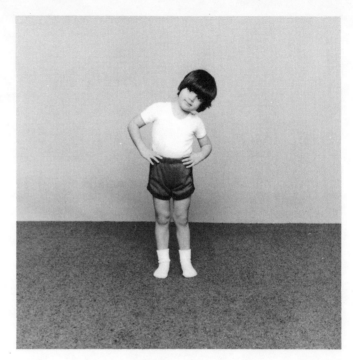

Figure 70

2. Tilt head to the right, then to the left. *(See figures 69 and 70.)*

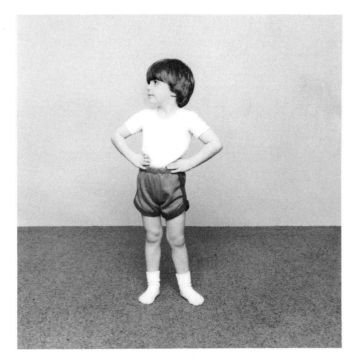
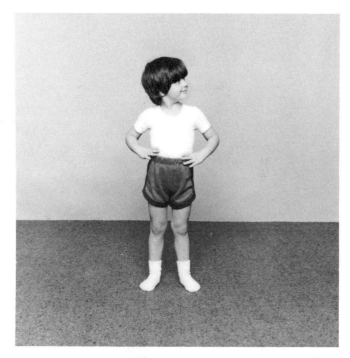

Figure 71　　　　　　　　　　　　**Figure 72**

3. Turn head to the right, then to the left. *(See figures 71 and 72.)*

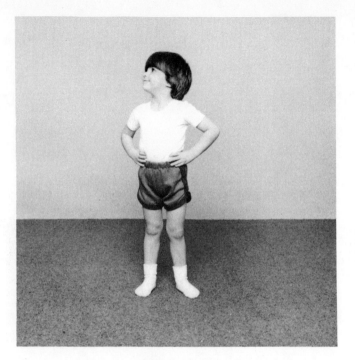

Figure 73

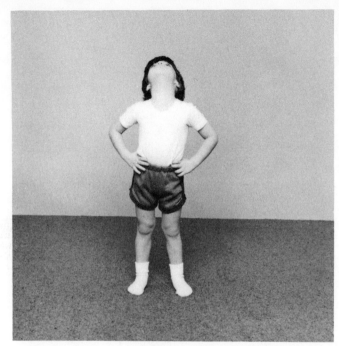

Figure 74

4. Rotate head slowly to the right three times, then slowly to the left three times. *(See figures 73 and 74.)*

FOR THE TRUNK

(These exercises are important for improving the mobility and tone of the vertebral column and in preventing lordorsis—forward curvature of the lower spine. Since at this age the musculature of the stomach and back is not very strong, keep the exercises brief and not too vigorous at the start.)

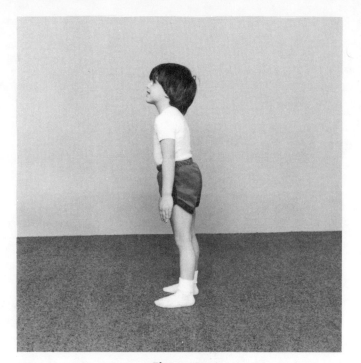
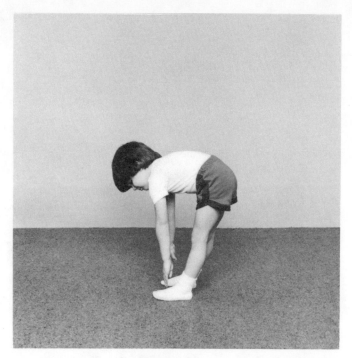

Figure 75   **Figure 76**

1. Stand with hands at the sides. Bend forward, try to touch the toes, and return. *(See figures 75 and 76.)*

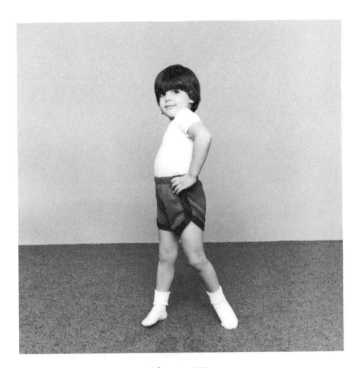

Figure 77

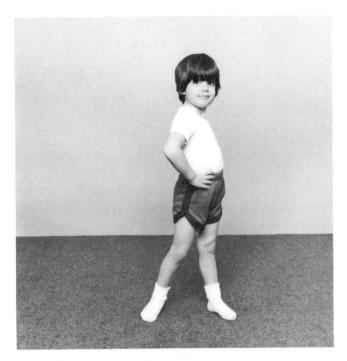

Figure 78

2. Stand with legs apart and hands on hips. Twist body to the right, then to the left. *(See figures 77 and 78.)*

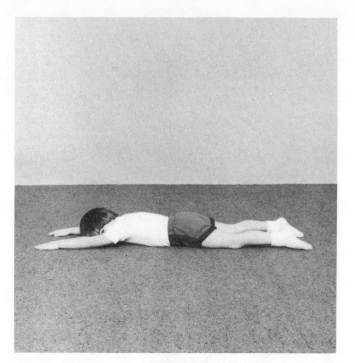

Figure 79

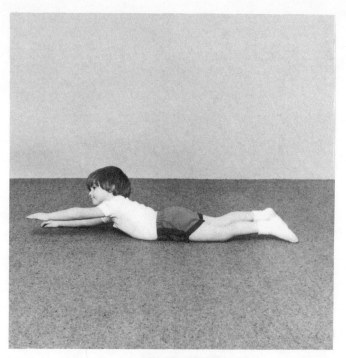

Figure 80

3. Lie on stomach with arms extended in front of head. Raise right arm and lower it, then left. *(See figures 79 and 80.)*

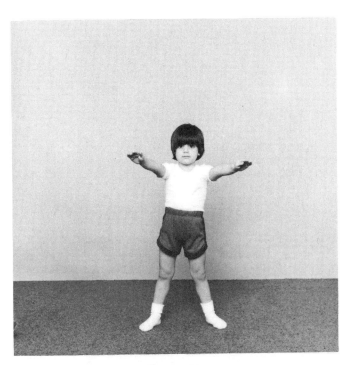

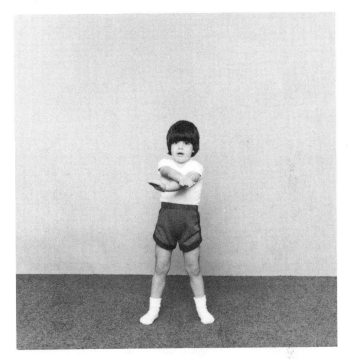

Figure 81   **Figure 82**

4. Stand with legs apart, arms in front. Keeping arms straight, scissor them briskly back and forth in front of the body. *(See figures 81 and 82.)*

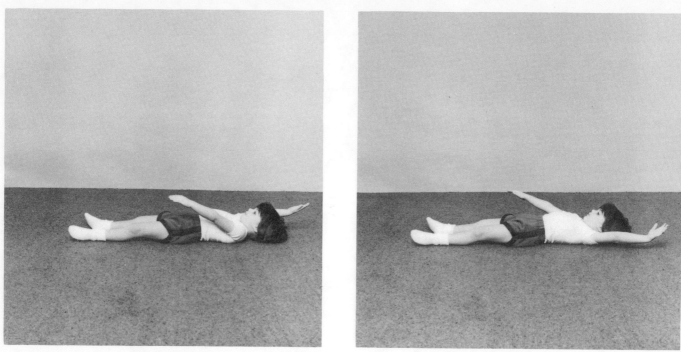

Figure 83 **Figure 84**

5. Lying on the back, extend the right arm overhead with the left at the side. Scissor them. *(See figures 83 and 84.)*

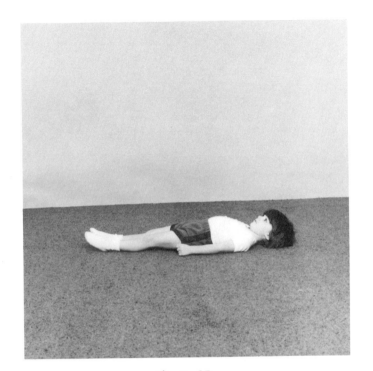

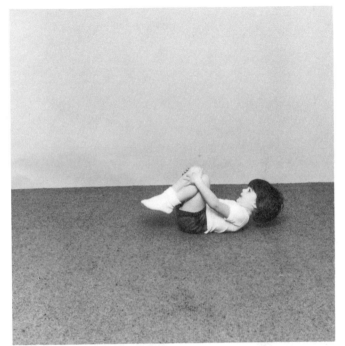

Figure 85

Figure 86

6. Lying on the back, lift knees to the chest and touch them with the hands. *(See figures 85 and 86.)*

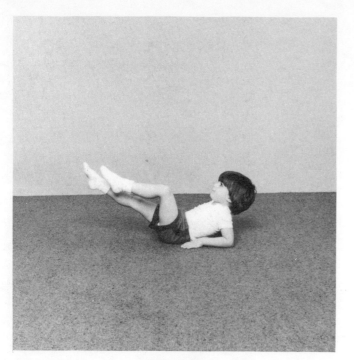

Figure 87

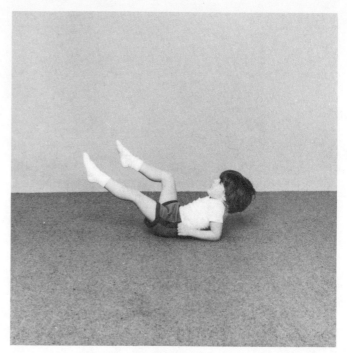

Figure 88

7. Sit on the floor, leaning back and supporting the body on elbows and palms. Lift the legs and pedal an imaginary bicycle for a count of ten. *(See figures 87 and 88.)*

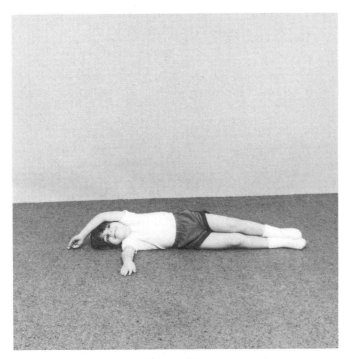

Figure 89

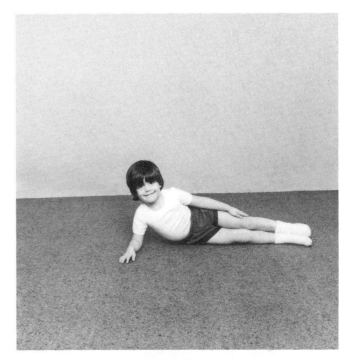

Figure 90

8. Lie on the right side, with right arm extended in front of body and left arm on floor above the head. Sit up by pressing with right arm and try to touch toes with left hand. Alternate on the left side. *(See figures 89 and 90.)*

FOR THE LEGS

(Strong, straight legs not only determine how well we walk and run but also greatly influence the body's posture and grace. Go beyond these exercises to encourage their use: Jump and skip and have impromptu races when you're out for a walk.)

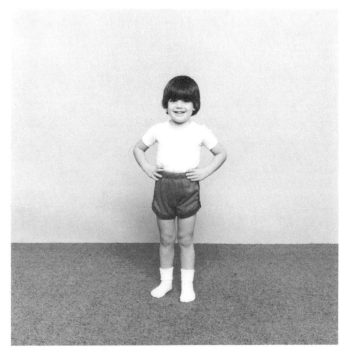

Figure 91

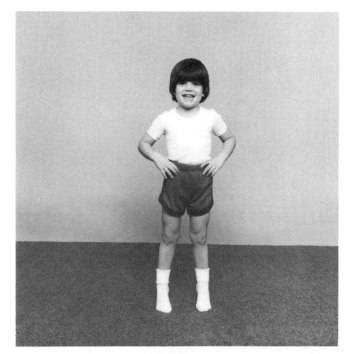

Figure 92

1. Stand with feet together, rise on the toes, and down. *(See figures 91 and 92.)*

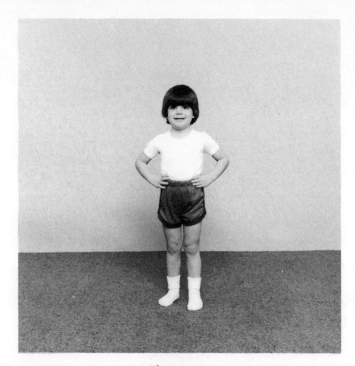

Figure 93

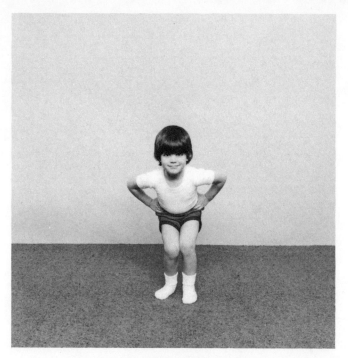

Figure 94

2. Stand with hands on hips, make a half knee bend, and straighten. *(See figures 93 and 94.)*

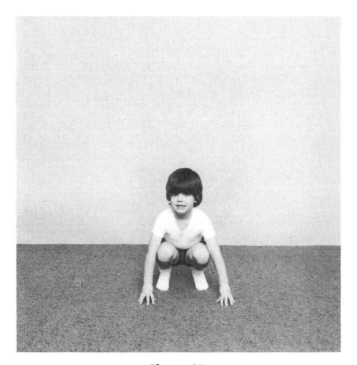

Figure 95

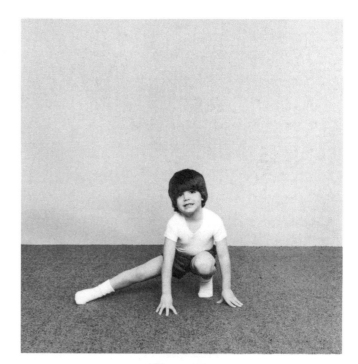

Figure 96

3. Squat on the floor, supporting body with the hands. Extend the right leg to the side and return, then do the same with the left leg. *(See figures 95 and 96.)*

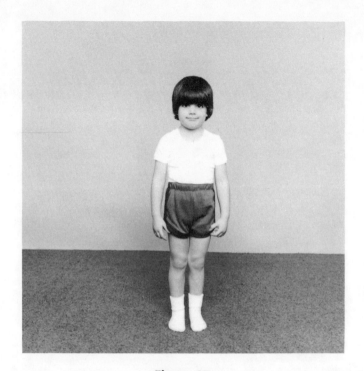

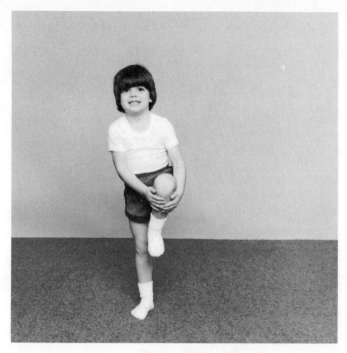

Figure 97   **Figure 98**

4. Stand with legs together and arms at the sides. Raise left leg and grasp it with both hands, pull to chest. Repeat with right leg. *(See figures 97 and 98.)*

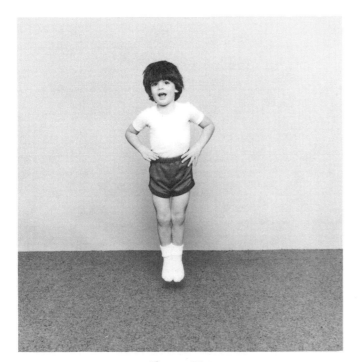

Figure 99

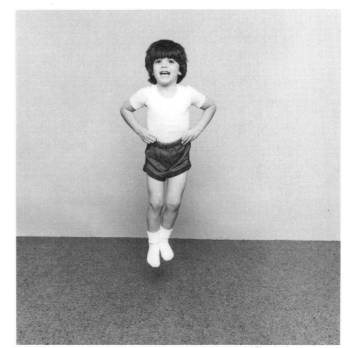

Figure 100

5. Stand with legs together, hands on hips. Jump lightly in place. *(See figures 99 and 100.)*

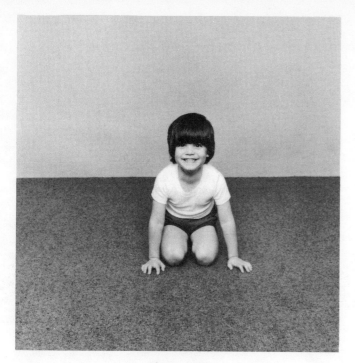

Figure 101

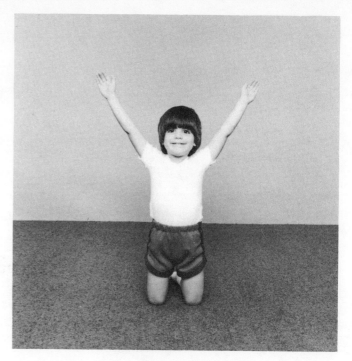

Figure 102

6. Kneel with palms on the floor, sitting on heels. Raise torso and arms up, then back to kneeling position. *(See figures 101 and 102.)*

Chapter IV

AGE FIVE TO EIGHT

As these years begin, you realize that you no longer have a baby. Your child is less dependent on you, both physically and emotionally, and more in tune with the outside world. He or she is starting the great adventure of school and is adjusting to discipline and group play. During these three years, the child usually is balanced and stable, welcoming the new demands on himself or herself—unless they come too quickly.

This means that in your exercise sessions you will find that young students now have the potential to understand and prize the goals you are aiming at. They begin to be aware that there is value, particularly among their schoolmates, in being able to run fast, climb a jungle gym, or throw a ball well. Now it will pay for you to explain—briefly and simply—what each exercise is designed to accomplish. When they start watching sports on TV, see if they can spot the specific abilities of a quarterback, a pitcher, a tennis player, and help them to relate these skills to their exercises.

If you haven't already done so, I recommend that you start at the beginning of these years to teach your child to know left from right—an accomplishment that he or she will be proud of and that will lighten your load in directing exercises. My second recommendation is that you begin, in easy stages, to get the child used to preparing the exercise area, so that by seven the student is handling that chore alone.

The point of this is much more than simply to

free you from a boring task. As I said earlier, exercises have a value far beyond the development of a strong, healthy body; they demonstrate to the growing child that effort—sometimes strenuous effort—is needed to produce worthwhile results.

All of us must learn the truth of that old line, "There is no such thing as a free lunch." Exercises are a great way to start teaching that lesson, and then it is up to the parent to broaden the child's area of responsibility.

WARM-UP

As always, each session must start with a brief warm-up period to prepare your child both physically and psychologically for the more strenuous efforts ahead. Begin by walking briskly (in place if necessary) ten paces each on the toes, on the heels, and on the outsides of the feet. Then run ten paces with the knees straight, lifting feet in front, and ten lifting feet to rear. Skip ten times. Jump in place ten times, scissoring legs alternately front and back. Now, standing with legs apart, stretch the arms to the sides and rotate them. Bring them in front and scissor them up and down. With arms overhead, rotate the trunk, five times to the right, five to the left. Then sit, with legs apart and arms overhead. Stretch and touch the right toes, then the left, five times each. Still sitting, complete the warm-up by bracing the hands on the floor behind the shoulders and raising the body on hands and heels ten times.

Keep the warm-up short—under five minutes—and lively, so it doesn't bore your child. But remember, it is essential in readying the body and avoiding strained muscles later. You can make it more fun by speeding up, then slowing down to slow motion.

82

FOR THE ARMS

(The goal is to improve coordination as well as flexibility, strength, and speed.)

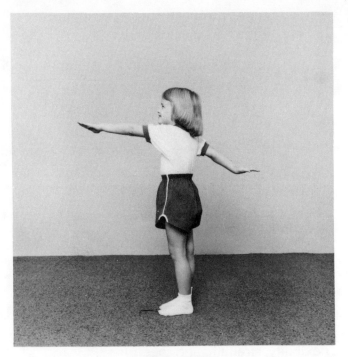

Figure 103

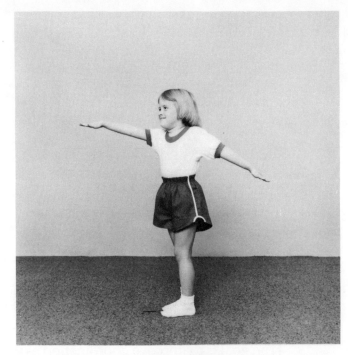

Figure 104

1. Standing with legs together, bring the left arm forward and up while swinging the right arm back; then reverse. *(See figures 103 and 104.)*

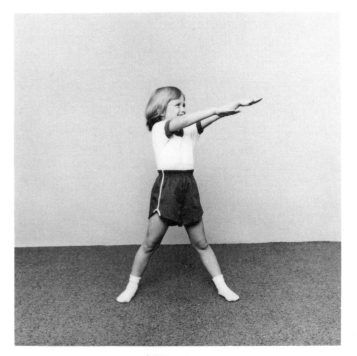

Figure 105

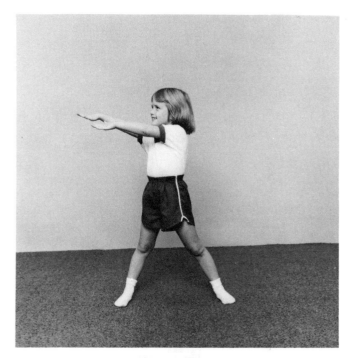

Figure 106

2. Stand with legs apart, holding both arms to the left at shoulder level. Swing them down in a semicircle and up to shoulder level on the right; then swing to the left. *(See figures 105 and 106.)*

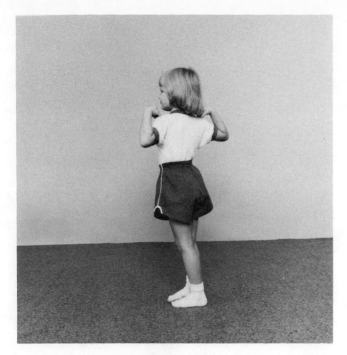

Figure 107

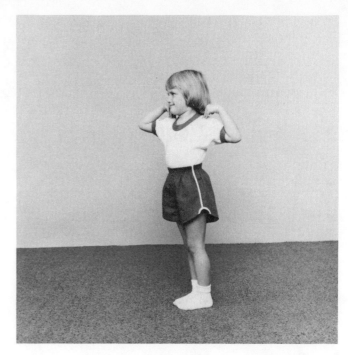

Figure 108

3. Standing with hands on shoulders, rotate the left shoulder forward and the right back; then alternate. *(See figures 107 and 108.)*

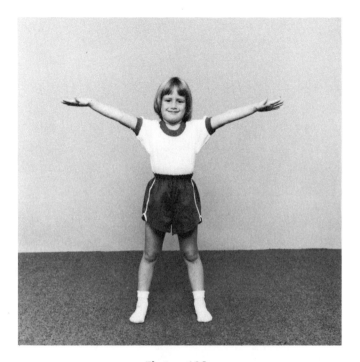

Figure 109

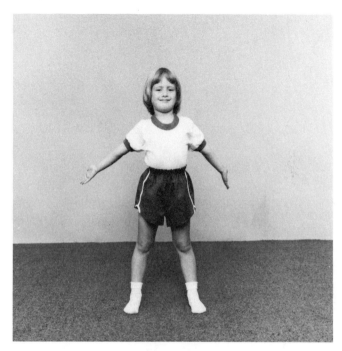

Figure 110

4. Stand with legs apart and arms thrust forward at shoulder level. Rotate arms in large circles, first in one direction, then in the opposite direction for thirty seconds. *(See figures 109 and 110.)*

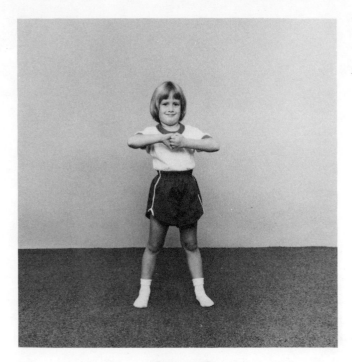

Figure 111

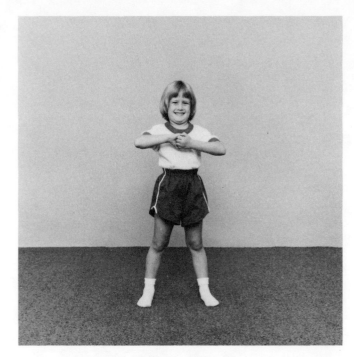

Figure 112

5. Clasp hands in front of chest with legs apart and elbows out to the sides. Pull hard, then relax. *(See figures 111 and 112.)*

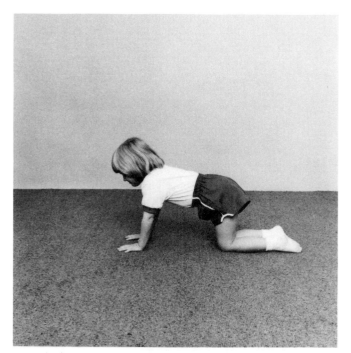

Figure 113

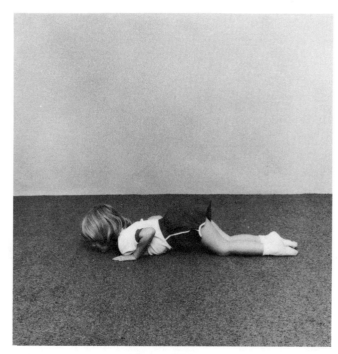

Figure 114

6. Kneel, supporting body with palms and knees. Do six push-ups. *(See figures 113 and 114.)*

FOR THE NECK

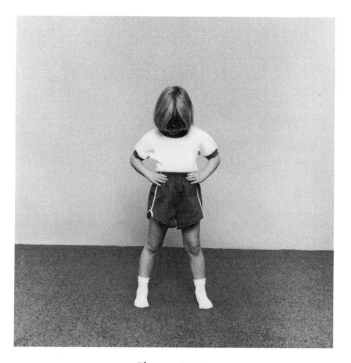

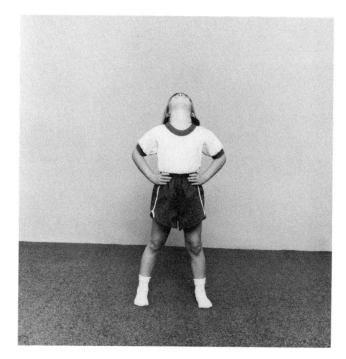

Figure 115   **Figure 116**

1. Bend head down to the chest and then arch backward. *(See figures 115 and 116.)*

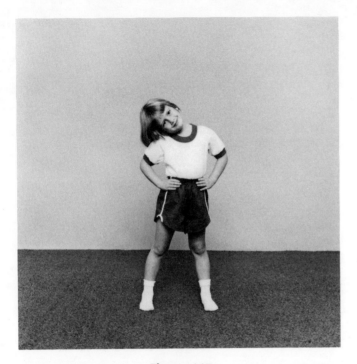

Figure 117

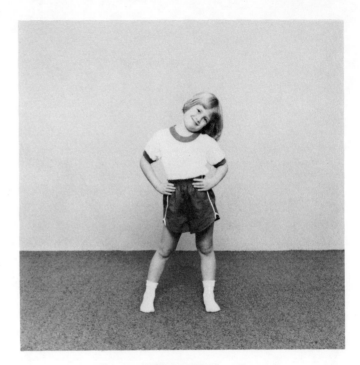

Figure 118

2. Tilt head to the right, then to the left. *(See figures 117 and 118.)*

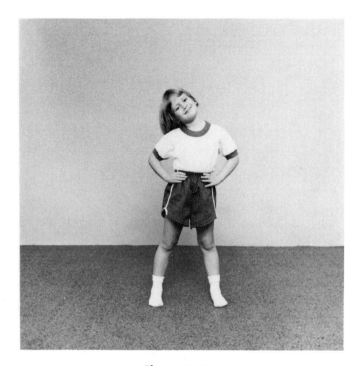

Figure 119

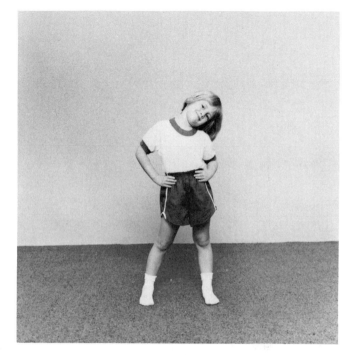

Figure 120

3. Tilt head to the right, then to the left. *(See figures 119 and 120.)*

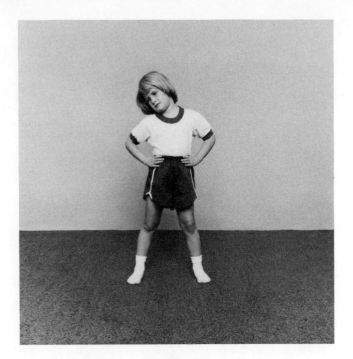

Figure 121

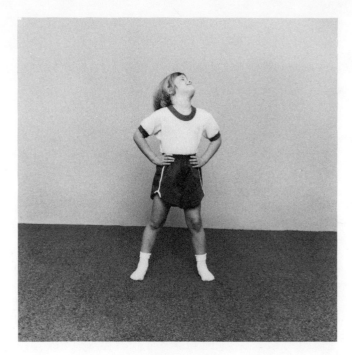

Figure 122

4. Rotate head slowly to the right three times, then slowly three times to the left. *(See figures 121 and 122.)*

FOR THE TRUNK

(These exercises are designed to strengthen the back and stomach muscles, which help maintain good posture by providing firm support for the spinal column. Remind your child to contract the stomach muscles and keep the lower back on the floor while doing those exercises that require lying on the back.)

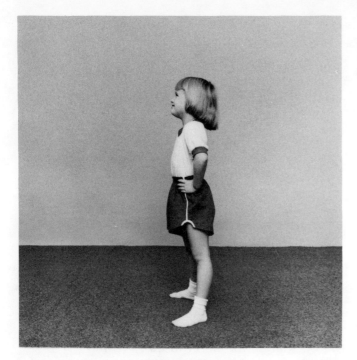

Figure 123

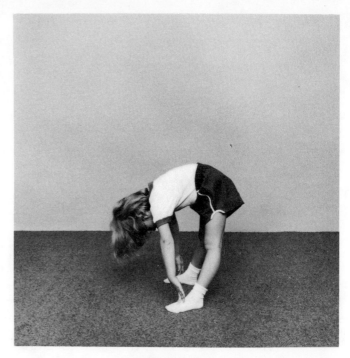

Figure 124

1. Stand with feet apart and hands on hips. Bend forward and touch toes, and return. *(See figures 123 and 124.)*

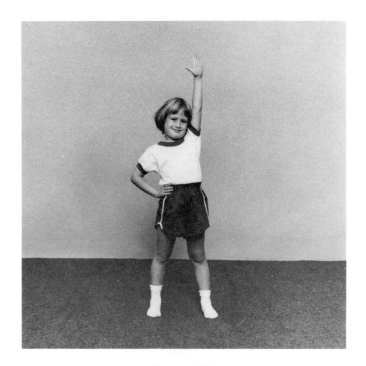
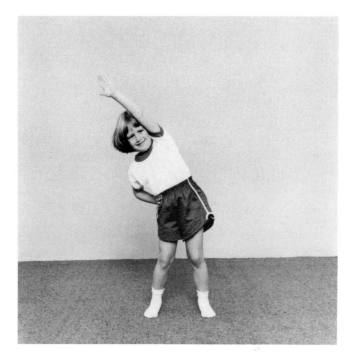

Figure 125   **Figure 126**

2. Stand with feet apart, right hand on hip and left hand overhead. Bend body to the right and return, twice. Then change arms and bend body twice to the left. *(See figures 125 and 126.)*

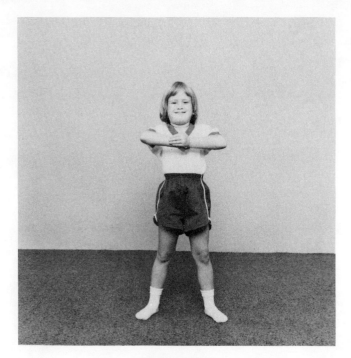

Figure 127

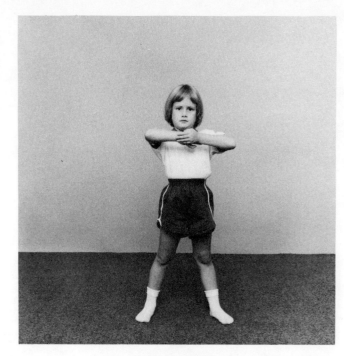

Figure 128

3. Stand with feet apart and hands clasped, palm to palm, in front of chest. Push together firmly, then relax. *(See figures 127 and 128.)*

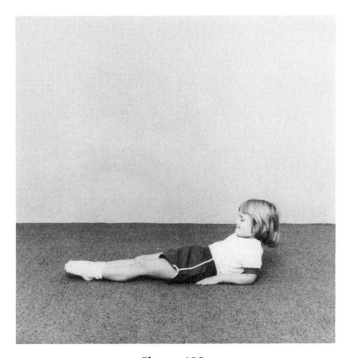

Figure 129

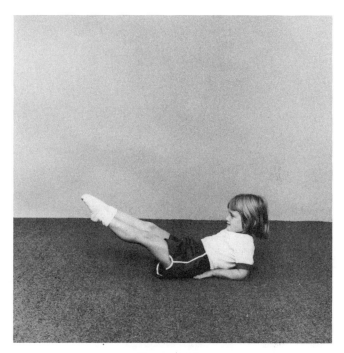

Figure 130

4. In reclining position, leaning back on elbows and forearms, raise legs at a 45-degree angle to the floor. Keeping them straight, execute a scissors movement vertically, then horizontally. *(See figures 129 and 130.)*

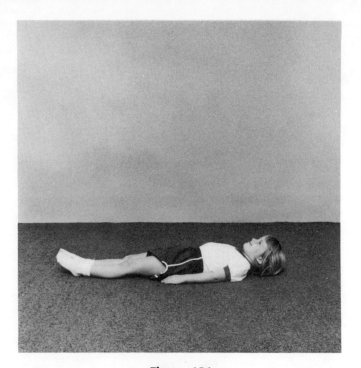

Figure 131

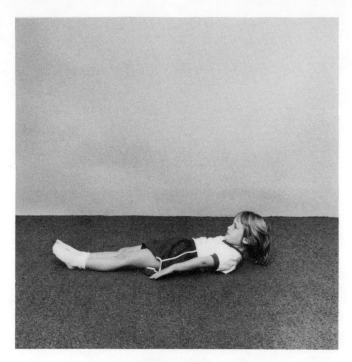

Figure 132

5. Lie on the back with arms at sides. Raise the head and shoulders off the floor, then lower. *(See figures 131 and 132.)*

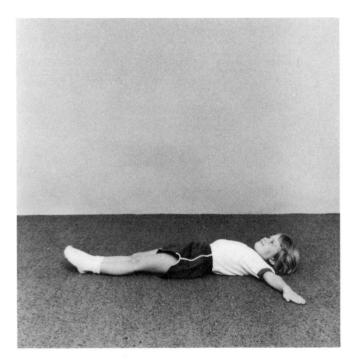

Figure 133

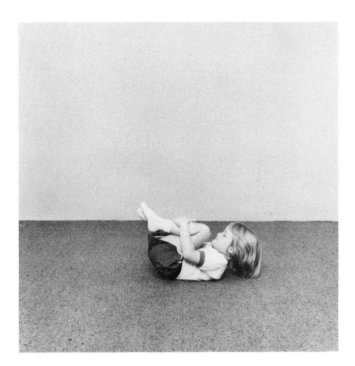

Figure 134

6. Lie on the back with arms out to the sides. Grasp knees with hands, pull them toward the chest, and bring the body to a sitting position. *(See figures 133 and 134.)*

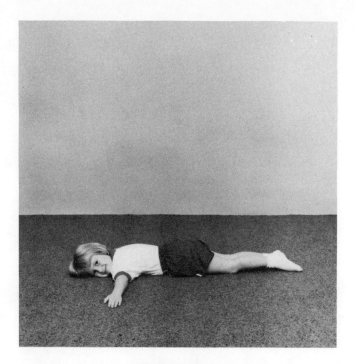

Figure 135

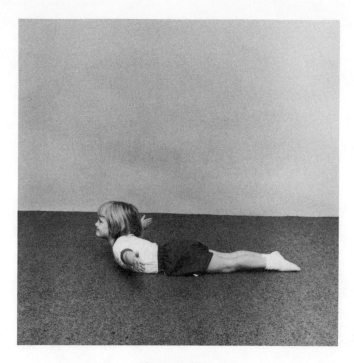

Figure 136

7. Lie on the stomach with arms out to the sides. Raise the head and chest while keeping legs on the floor. *(See figures 135 and 136.)*

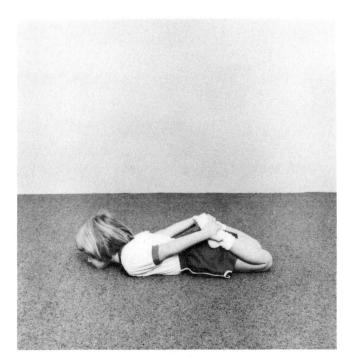

Figure 137

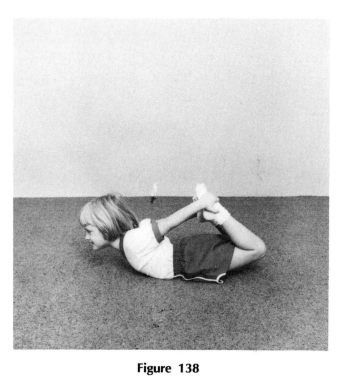

Figure 138

8. Lie on the stomach with knees bent. Grasp ankles in hands and arch back by pulling head and feet toward each other; then relax. *(See figures 137 and 138.)*

FOR THE LEGS

(This is the age to teach good walking habits: upright posture, smooth rhythm, with legs and opposite arms swinging forward freely. The running exercises here improve motor speed, and jumping is important in strengthening joints. Landings should be soft, on the balls of the feet, with ankle and leg joints flexing slightly to absorb the shock.)

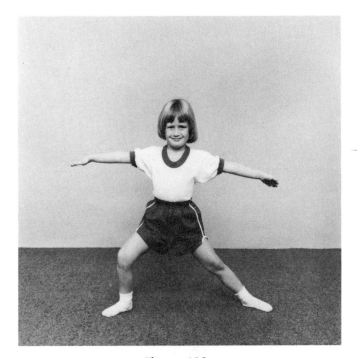

Figure 139

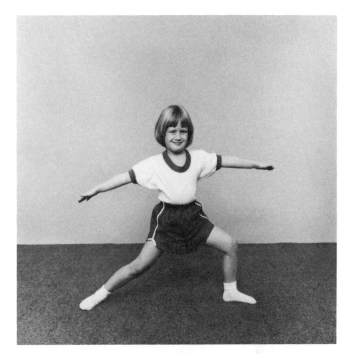

Figure 140

1. Take a fairly long step to the side with the right foot, bending the right knee and raising hands to shoulder height. Return, and do the same to the left. *(See figures 139 and 140.)*

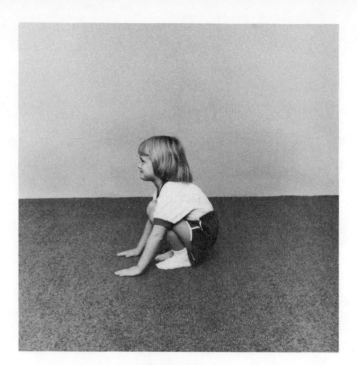

Figure 141

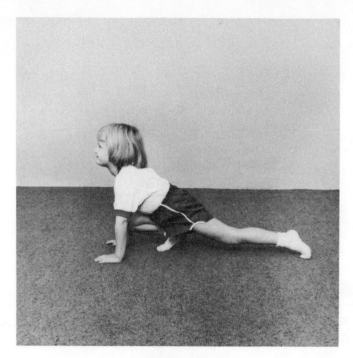

Figure 142

2. In a squatting position, with hands on floor, thrust left leg back and return, then right leg. *(See figures 141 and 142.)*

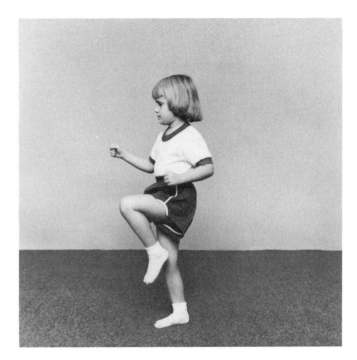

Figure 143

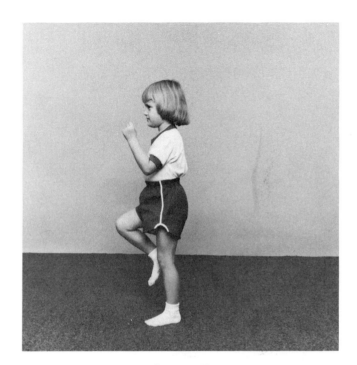

Figure 144

3. Run in place, raising the knees toward the chest on each stride. *(See figures 143 and 144.)*

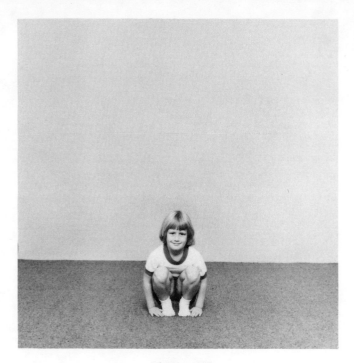

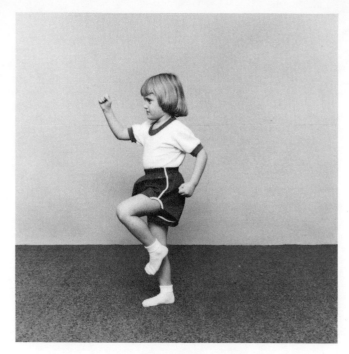

Figure 145   **Figure 146**

4. While your child is running easily in place, clap your hands as a signal for him or her to jump up lightly and land in a squat, then spring up immediately and continue running. *(See figures 145 and 146.)*

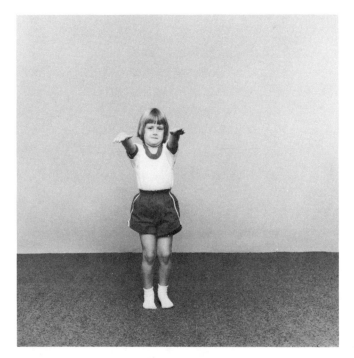

Figure 147

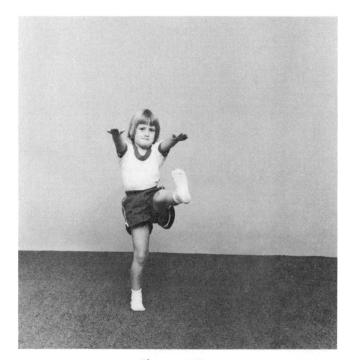

Figure 148

5. Stand with feet together and arms in front at shoulder level. Kick left leg toward right hand, then right leg toward left hand. *(See figures 147 and 148.)*

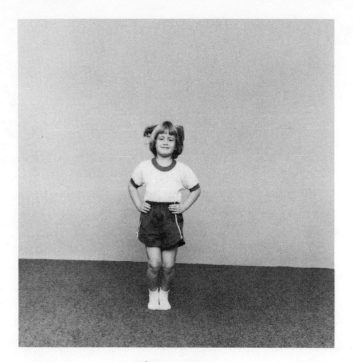

Figure 149

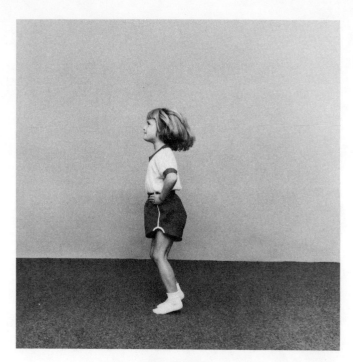

Figure 150

6. With hands on hips, jump three times in place. Make the fourth jump higher, turn 90 degrees to the right, and land. Do the same to the left. *(See figures 149 and 150.)*

Chapter V

AGE EIGHT THROUGH ELEVEN

There will be times now when your child seems almost grown-up. Motor skills have improved, and you will realize that the exercise program has led to fluid, graceful body movements. Since children of this age have the capacity to understand the value of each exercise, they will probably participate more enthusiastically, too.

This leads to a cautionary note: During these years, children often have an intense desire to perfect various skills, whether it be the multiplication table or push-ups. You must keep in mind that they still are children and should not exhaust themselves. Their arms and legs are growing at a rate that foreshadows the growth spurt of adolescence; and muscles, including the heart, are not keeping up. Although they appear to be rugged, don't make the mistake of treating children of this age like trained athletes. Don't let them exceed the schedule of exercises, and see to it that they take a breather between strenuous sets.

If the earlier years of exercise have gone reasonably well, you have all the more reason to expect your child's ready cooperation during this period. He or she is eager to learn and also likes to spend time with mother or father. Your support and praise is still needed, but you no longer have to do the exercises with your child—just demonstrate the movements and set the rhythm. It's true that children this age like a contest, whether with their peers or with a parent, and if you're in shape you can accept their challenges—but I don't urge it.

One last suggestion: Encourage your child to play outdoors with friends—running, wrestling, jumping, climbing, throwing. These activities will consolidate and use the muscle skills learned in the systematic exercise program.

WARM-UP

Walk in place, rolling from the heels to the toes at a faster and faster pace until it becomes running. After one minute, stop, raise arms up from the sides, and inhale, down and exhale, four times. Now do ten jumps, twisting first to the right, then to the left, landing lightly on the toes.

Starting with arms overhead, turn trunk to the right and touch the right toe, then up and repeat to the left, five times to each side. Hold arms out to the sides and twist the trunk right and left ten times. With arms in front and legs together, kick each foot to the hands five times. Finally, with legs wide apart and hands on knees, bend the right knee, twisting the trunk to the right, then alternate to the left, ten times.

FOR THE ARMS

(These exercises concentrate on developing strength and coordination. Some are strenuous—particularly the push-ups and the isometrics, where one muscle strains against another. It's important for your child to have a rest period between them; urge deep breathing with emphasis on exhaling strongly. "Blow the old air out, the way a whale does.")

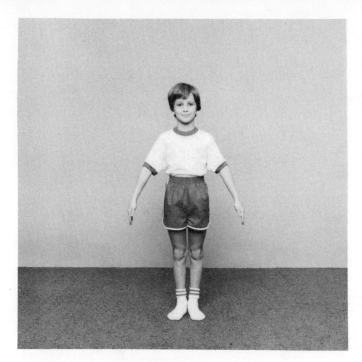

Figure 151

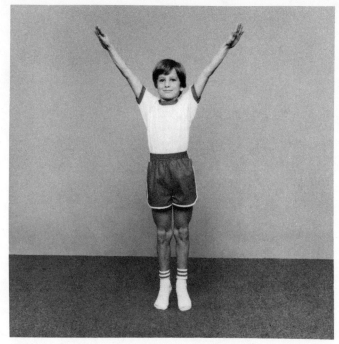

Figure 152

1. Stand with arms at sides. Extend them in one motion to the sides and overhead while rising on the toes; then lower. *(See figures 151 and 152.)*

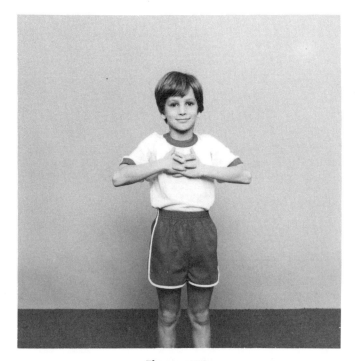

Figure 153

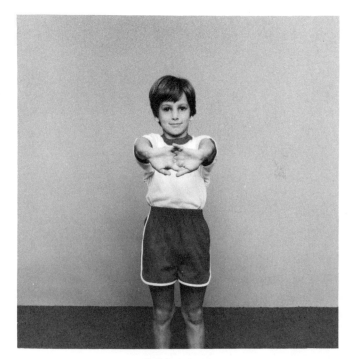

Figure 154

2. Stand with legs apart and interlace fingers on front of chest. Turn palms out and straighten arms. *(See figures 153 and 154.)*

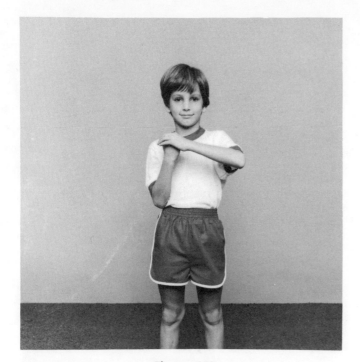

Figure 155

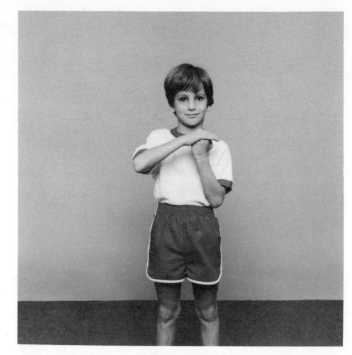

Figure 156

3. Stand with arms bent—the right elbow pointed down, the left out to the side. Cup the left hand over the right fist and try to raise the right arm, while holding it down with the left, for five to seven seconds. Repeat with opposite hands. Then give young muscles a rest. *(See figures 155 and 156.)*

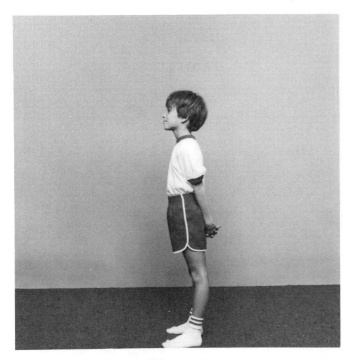

Figure 157

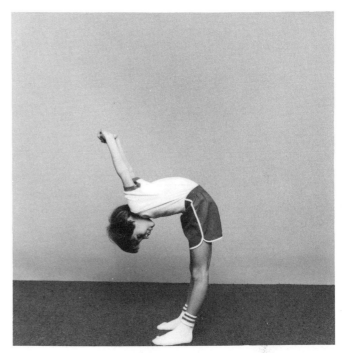

Figure 158

4. Stand with the hands clasped in back. Raise the hands backward while bending the body forward toward the knees. *(See figures 157 and 158.)*

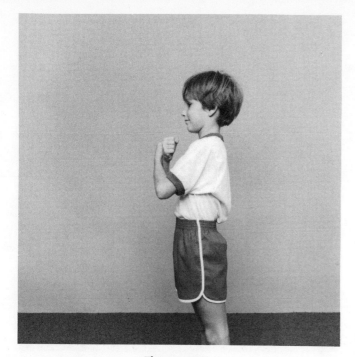

Figure 159

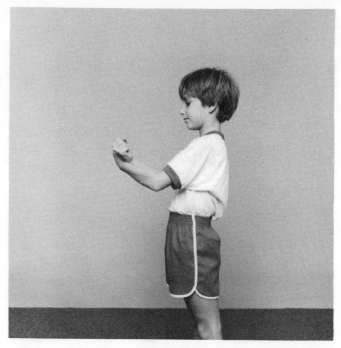

Figure 160

5. Cross arms in front of body, with hands making fists. Press out with inside arm while holding it in with the other for five to seven seconds. Then reverse arms and repeat. Again, give muscles a rest. *(See figures 159 and 160.)*

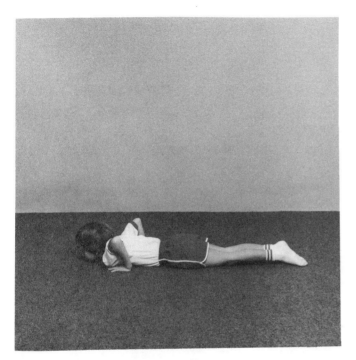

Figure 161

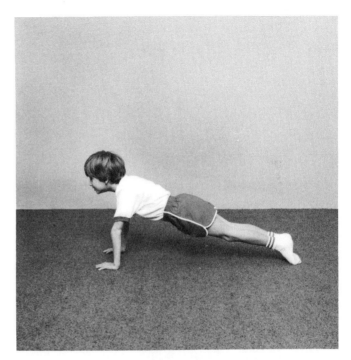

Figure 162

6. Lie prone, with palms on floor under shoulders. Push up, supporting body on palms and toes, keeping back straight; then lower body to the floor. Rest. *(See figures 161 and 162.)*

FOR THE NECK

(Now the neck is strong enough to perform its limited movements against resistance.)

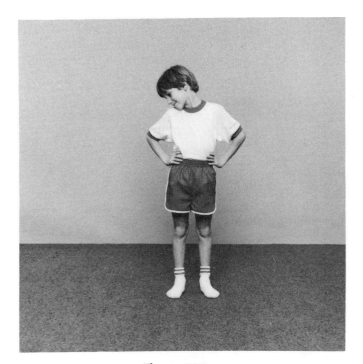

Figure 163

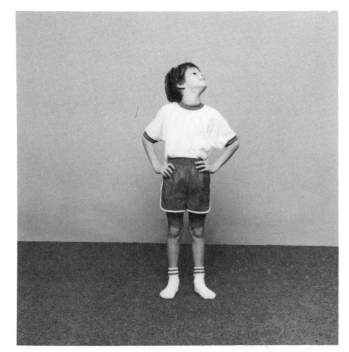

Figure 164

1. Tilt head to the right and rotate it slowly three times to the right. Then do the same to the left. This is a simple but important exercise; do not omit it. *(See figures 163 and 164.)*

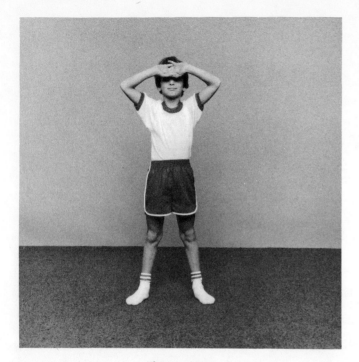

Figure 165

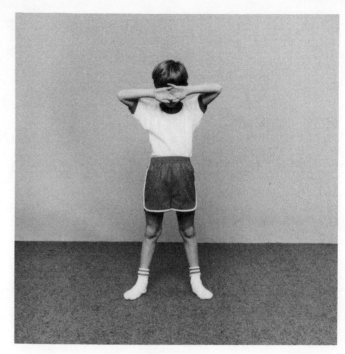

Figure 166

2. Clasp the hands and hold them against the forehead. Push the head forward against their resistance. *(See figures 165 and 166.)*

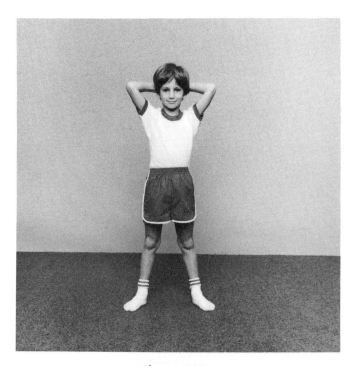

Figure 167

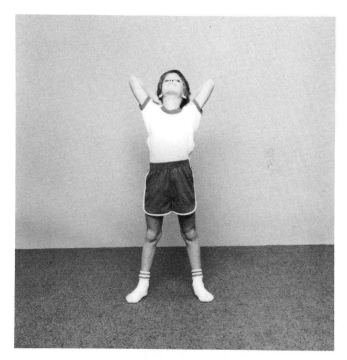

Figure 168

3. Clasp the hands behind the head and push back. *(See figures 167 and 168.)*

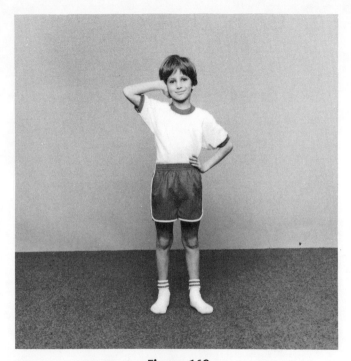

Figure 169

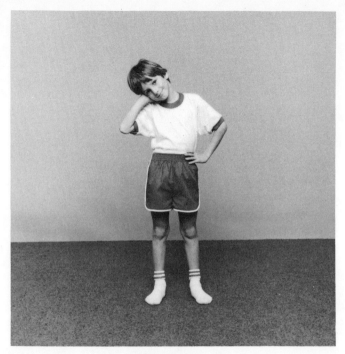

Figure 170

4. Place right palm on head over ear, with elbow out to the right side. Tilt head to the right against the hand's resistance. Repeat to the left side. *(See figures 169 and 170.)*

FOR THE TRUNK

(The first four of these exercises are designed to strengthen abdominal muscles, where most of us are weakest. In performing them, the back muscles should be used as little as possible. Now you can teach the breathing method that gymnasts use: Exhale strongly near the end of the most difficult part of the exercise; e.g., just before the legs touch the floor in Exercise 2.)

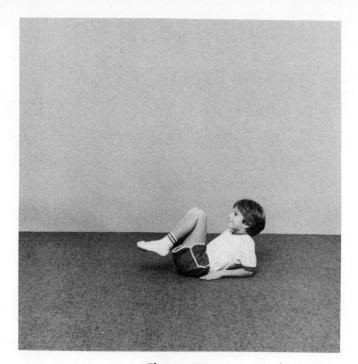

Figure 171

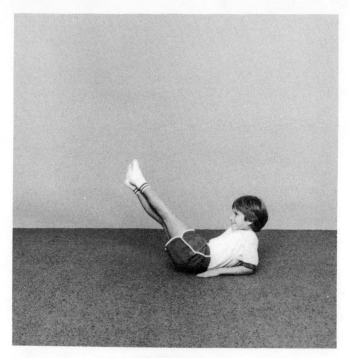

Figure 172

1. Sit on the floor with legs straight, leaning back on elbows. Bring the knees to the chest, straighten them out to the right at a 45-degree angle to the floor, return to chest, straighten them to the left, and return. *(See figures 171 and 172.)*

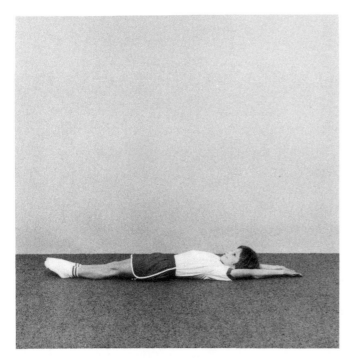

Figure 173

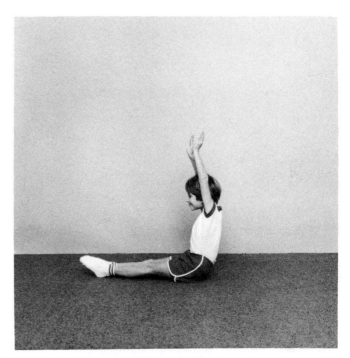

Figure 174

2. Lie on the back with arms overhead. Sit up slowly and pause briefly with the body in a vertical position, then slowly lower body back to the floor. Now bring the legs to a vertical position while keeping them straight, and slowly lower them to the floor. *(See figures 173 and 174.)*

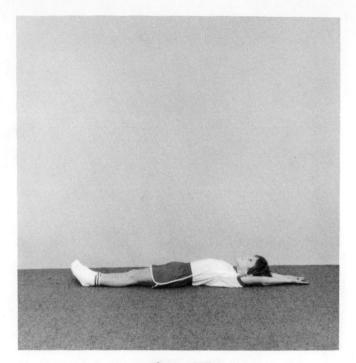

Figure 175

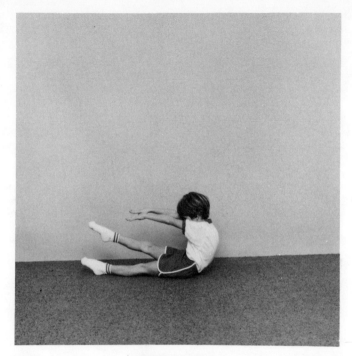

Figure 176

3. Lie on the back with arms overhead and "jackknife" with one leg—raise the right leg and upper body simultaneously, keeping both straight. Then do the same with the left leg. *(See figures 175 and 176.)*

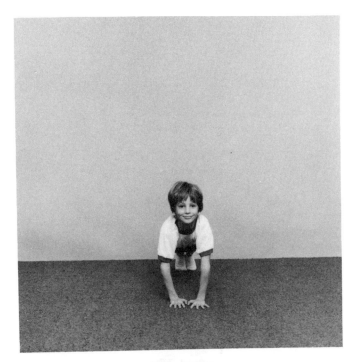

Figure 177

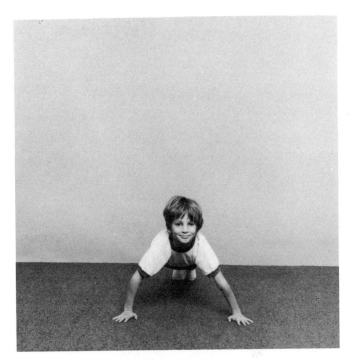

Figure 178

4. In push-up position, with body supported on palms and toes, slide palms out to the sides as far as possible while supporting the body, then slide hands back. *(See figures 177 and 178.)*

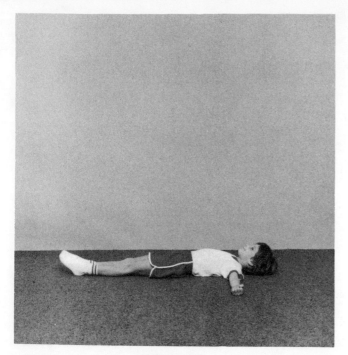

Figure 179

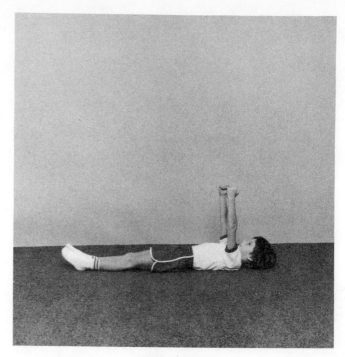

Figure 180

5. Lying on the back, extend arms to the sides, making fists. Bring up in front of chest, then back down. *(See figures 179 and 180.)*

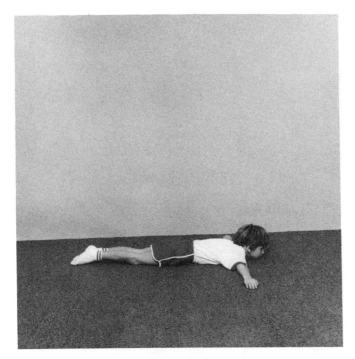

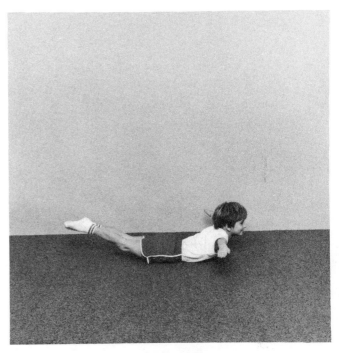

Figure 181   **Figure 182**

6. Lie on the stomach with arms out to the sides. Simultaneously lift arms, legs, head, and chest, then lower. *(See figures 181 and 182.)*

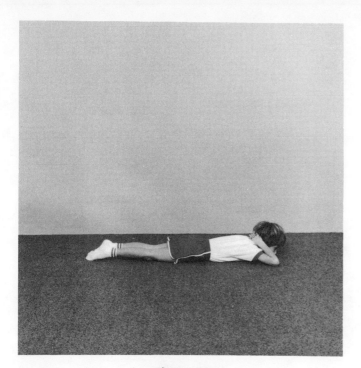

Figure 183

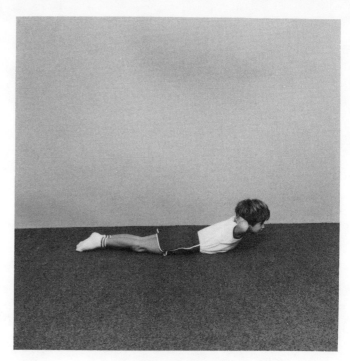

Figure 184

7. Lie on the stomach with hands clasped behind neck. Raise the upper body, twist to the right, and lower. Alternate to the left. *(See figures 183 and 184.)*

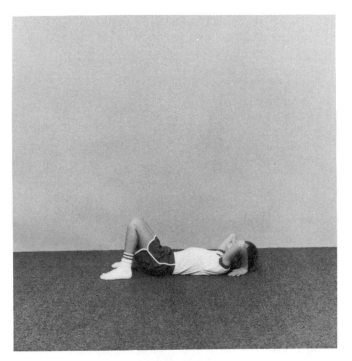

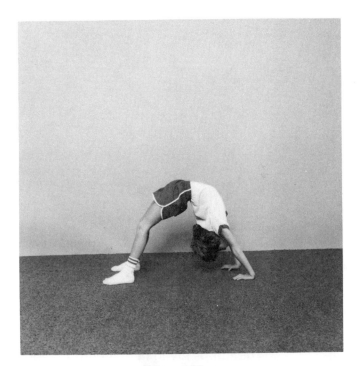

Figure 185   **Figure 186**

8. Lie on the back and raise trunk from floor with arms and legs. "Walk" hands toward feet until body is arched in a backbend. Lower slowly. *(See figures 185 and 186.)*

FOR THE LEGS

(The jumps given here are important for strengthening the muscles and articulations of the legs, but they must be performed correctly, with the legs flexed to act as shock absorbers on landing. "Land softly, like a cat.")

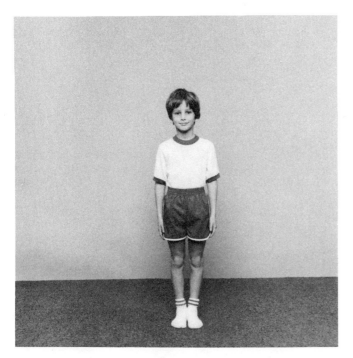

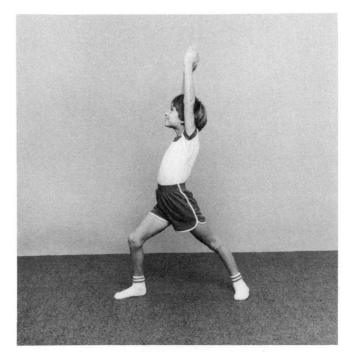

Figure 187   **Figure 188**

1. Stand with arms at sides. Turn the body to the right and take a long step with the right leg, swinging arms smoothly overhead while bending the right knee. Bring legs back together while swinging arms down, and repeat to the left. *(See figures 187 and 188.)*

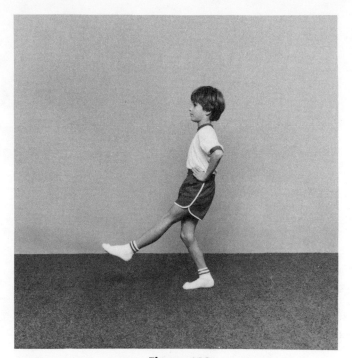

Figure 189

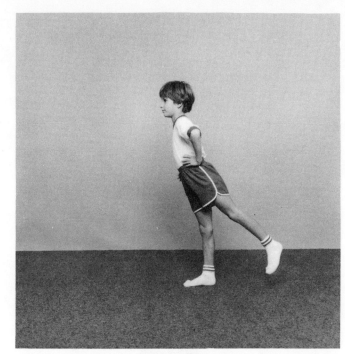

Figure 190

2. Jump on the right leg while swinging the left leg forward and back three times, then side to side three times. Alternate on the left leg. *(See figures 189 and 190.)*

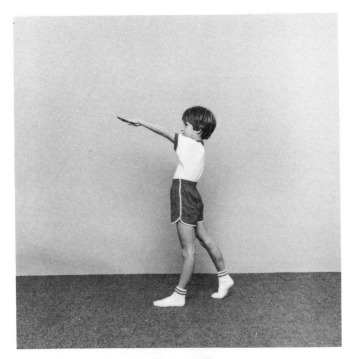

Figure 191

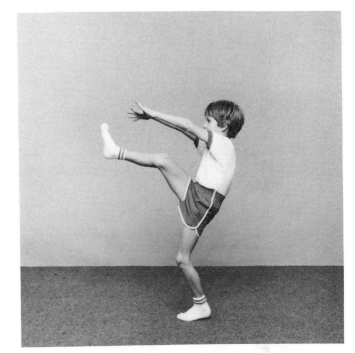

Figure 192

3. Stand with hands level with the head and weight advanced on the left leg. Jump up lightly on the left leg, kicking the right leg to hands. Alternate legs. *(See figures 191 and 192.)*

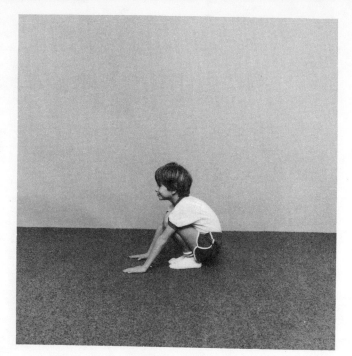

Figure 193

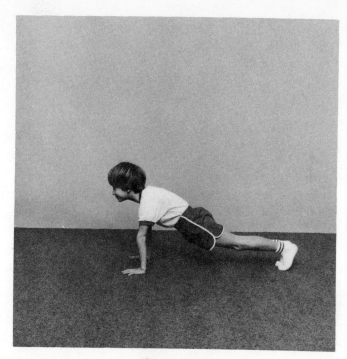

Figure 194

4. From a standing position, squat with palms on the floor. Jump with both legs straight back, return to squatting position, and stand up. *(See figures 193 and 194.)*

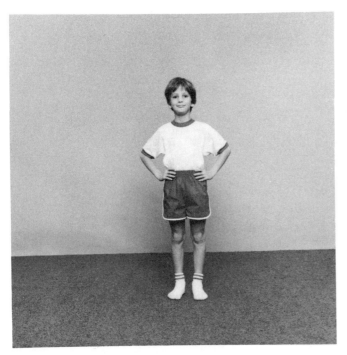

Figure 195

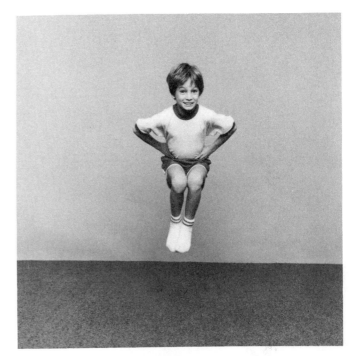

Figure 196

5. Stand with hands on hips, jumping easily in place. Every fourth jump, raise the knees to the chest—and land lightly! *(See figures 195 and 196.)*

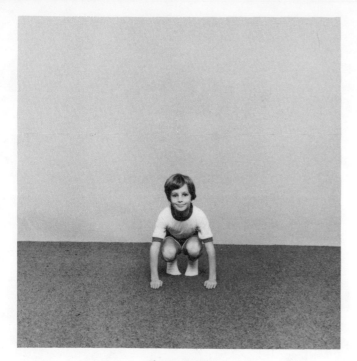

Figure 197

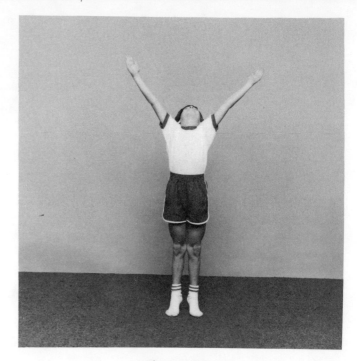

Figure 198

6. From a squatting position, jump high in the air with legs together and arms spread, reaching to the sky. Land back in a squatting position. *(See figures 197 and 198.)*

ABOUT THE AUTHOR

Radu Teodorescu is one of the fortunate few who make their living by doing what they most enjoy —in his case, exercising. When he is not briskly directing the workouts of such glamorous clients as Halston, Bianca Jagger, Joel Schumacher, and Angelo Donghia in his Manhattan studio, he is acting as teacher and athletic coach in a private school or giving exercise tips to television audiences. Characteristically, Radu never simply describes an exercise, he demonstrates it vigorously. His weekends are spent jogging or playing tennis or skiing, both with and without students.

Radu was born in Pitesti, Rumania, in 1944. After graduation from high school, where he showed outstanding athletic ability, he was drafted, but as soon as he completed his tour of duty he was accepted as a student by the Physical Culture Institute in Bucharest, having rated seventh-highest of 1100 candidates. He earned his bachelor's and master's degrees there and taught gymnastics on both the high-school and college level, and competed in national soccer and gymnastics teams.

In 1972 Radu escaped into Western Europe and arrived in the United States on his twenty-eighth birthday. He taught in several exercise studios in New York, then opened his own in 1977. He particularly enjoys working with children— "they don't have as many bad habits as the rest of us"—and this book was foreshadowed by a television mini-series on exercises for mothers and children that Radu originated and starred in.